Foreword

Cardiology is unique among medical specialties in three respects. First, it is the largest of all of the specialties. Cardiovascular disease is the most common cause of mortality and serious morbidity, being responsible for more than 40% of all deaths in the industrially developed nations, and the incidence is now rising rapidly in developing countries as well. Second, advances have been more rapid in cardiology than in the other medical specialties. All aspects of cardiology – prevention, diagnosis, pharmacologic and invasive therapy – have progressed at dizzying speeds during the past 20 years. Finally, cardiology is the clinical specialty that is most dependent on visual recognition. Beginning with the introduction of the electrocardiogram and chest roentgenogram at the turn of the 20th century to the development of a variety of sophisticated non-invasive techniques as we turn into the 21st century, the practice of cardiovascular medicine has always required the recognition of graphic waveforms and visual images.

This *Self-Assessment Color Review of Cardiology* recognizes all three unique aspects of the specialty. It is both broad and deep, and deals with all of the common and many of the uncommon cardiac disorders. I found the inclusion of the cardiovascular manifestations of disorders that affect other organ systems, as well as cardiac diseases observed most frequently in developing countries, to be particularly welcome.

This book achieves a good balance between classic time-honored clinical presentations of disease on the one hand and the most up-to-date diagnostic and therapeutic modalities on the other. The very high quality and diversity of the images and the valuable insights provided by the brief but pointed discussions make learning cardiology from this book an experience that is, at one time, intellectually invigorating, efficient and pleasant.

Eugene Braunwald, MD
Harvard Medical School
Brigham & Women's Hospital
Massachussetts General Hospital

Acknowledgements

Many colleagues, past and present, have been very generous in making available several of the illustrations shown. The authors would like to thank Ms Beverley Andrews, Dr John Axford, Dr Kanran Baig, Professor Stephen Bloom, Dr Laura Corr, Dr Graham Davies, Dr David Dutka, Dr Farzin Fath-Ordoubadi, Dr Rodney Foale, Professor John Goodwin, Professor Michael Hughes, Mr Lee Lewis, Ms Barbara Morgan, Dr Petros Nihoyannopoulos, Dr Peter Nixon, Professor Mark Noble, Dr Dinah Parums, Dr Ariela Pomerance, Mr Peter Smith, Professor Gilbert Thompson and Professor Richard Underwood. The advice of Dr Steve Hearne of Duke University Medical Center is also gratefully acknowledged, as is the New England Journal of Medicine's kind permission to reproduce Dr Naiman's beautiful photograph of *Digitalis purpurea* (*N Eng J Med* 1994; **331**: 1563).

Finally the authors would like to express their thanks to Professor Eugene Braunwald for doing them the honour of writing the foreword to this book.

Self-Assessment Color Review of
Cardiology

Stuart D. Rosen
MA, MRCP
MRC Clinical Scientist and
Hon Lecturer and Senior Registrar in Cardiology
Royal Postgraduate Medical School
Hammersmith Hospital, London

Sanjay Sharma
BSc (Hons), MRCP
Research Fellow in Cardiology
St George's Hospital Medical School, London
Lecturer for MEDIPASS

Celia M. Oakley
MD, FRCP
Professor of Clinical Cardiology
Royal Postgraduate Medical School
Hammersmith Hospital, London

With a Foreword by
Eugene Braunwald
Distinguished Hersey Professor of Medicine
Harvard Medical School
Faculty Dean for Academic Programs
Brigham & Women's Hospital and
Massachusetts General Hospital

LITTLE, BROWN AND COMPANY
Boston New York Toronto

To Ann, Seema and Ron

This edition published in the United States by:
Little, Brown and Company, 34 Beacon Street,
Boston, Massachusetts 02108–1493, 1997.
ISBN 0–316–75813–2
Available from Lippincott/Raven Publishers, Philadelphia

ISBN 1–874545–05–7

A CIP catalogue record for this book is available from the British Library.

Design and layout: Patrick Daly
Text editing: John Ormiston
Color reproduction: Tenon & Polert Colour Scanning Ltd, Hong Kong
Printed by: Grafos SA, Barcelona, Spain

Preface

Cardiology is one of the most important components of internal medicine and even the non-specialist must have a good working knowledge of it. For this reason, there has been and will continue to be a strong emphasis upon cardiology in postgraduate medical examinations such as the Membership of the Royal Colleges of Physicians in the United Kingdom and the Boards examinations in the United States. Both increasingly incorporate slides and pictures of the type presented in this book, which we have written principally for doctors in training who are approaching postgraduate examinations. We have tried to cover the broad sweep of adult cardiology (as well as some congenital heart disease) featured in the postgraduate curriculum and to include the ever-expanding range of cardiovascular investigations and imaging modalities. Because it is the purpose of our book to teach as well as to test, the answers are discursive. Some of the questions are based around investigations which are not in very common clinical usage today, such as M mode echocardiograms or even apexcardiograms; this has been a deliberate choice, because of the wealth of physiological and pathophysiological understanding which can be derived from them. Similarly, we have also presented a number of phonocardiograms, as this is the only obvious way to present auscultatory findings through the medium of a book. Being a self-assessment text, our book is not intended as a replacement for a standard cardiology textbook, but rather as a means of polishing and refining the reader's knowledge in readiness for an examination and identifying those areas of the subject in which further in-depth study is still necessary.

Cardiovascular disease remains one of the outstanding threats to human life and health. If you gain some greater cardiological expertise from reading this book, it will have served its purpose well.

Stuart D. Rosen
Royal Postgraduate Medical School
Hammersmith Hospital, London

Sanjay Sharma
St George's Hospital
Medical School, London

Celia M. Oakley
Royal Postgraduate Medical School
Hammersmith Hospital, London

Abbreviations

ACE – Angiotensin-converting enzyme
ADC – Apexcardiogram
AF – Atrial fibrillation
AICD – Automatic implantable cardioverter–defibrillator
AL – Amyloidosis
ANCA – Antineutrophil cytoplasmic antibodies
APBs – Atrial premature beats
APTT – Activated partial thromboplastin time
ASD – Atrial septal defect
ASO – Anti-streptolysin O
AST – Aspartate aminotransferase
AV – Atrioventricular
AVNRT – Atrioventricular nodal re-entrant tachycardia

BUN – Blood urea nitrogen

CABG – Coronary artery bypass grafting
CAD – Coronary artery disease
CCF – Congestive cardiac failure
CCU – Coronary Care Unit
CK – Creatine kinase
CPR – Cardiopulmonary resuscitation

DIC – Disseminated intravascular coagulation
DM – Diastolic murmur

ECG – Electrocardiogram
EMF – Endomyocardial fibrosis
ESR – Erythrocyte sedimentation rate

FA – Femoral artery
FBC – Full blood count
FDPs – Fibrin degradation products
FH – Familial hypercholesterolaemia
FSH – Follicle-stimulating hormone

HBD – Hydroxybutyric dehydrogenase
HCM – Hypertrophic cardiomyopathy
HDL – High density lipoprotein
HIV – Human immunodeficiency virus

IHSS – Idiopathic hypertrophic subaortic stenosis
INR – International normalised ratio

JVP – Jugular venous pressure

LAD – Left anterior descending coronary artery
LBBB – Left bundle branch block
LCA – Left coronary artery
LDH – Lactic dehydrogenase
LDL – Low density lipoprotein
LH – Luteinising hormone
LIMA – Left internal mammary artery
LSE – Left sternal edge
LV – Left ventricle
LVEDP – Left ventricular end-diastolic pressure
LVH – Left ventricular hypertrophy

MIBG – Metaiodobenzylguanidine
MRI – Magnetic resonance imaging
MUGA – Multi-gated ventriculogram

PTCA – Percutaneous transluminal coronary angioplasty

RBBB – Right bundle branch block
RVEDP – Right ventricular end-diastolic pressure

SLE – Systemic lupus erythematosus

T4 – Thyroxine
TGV – Transposition of great vessels
TOE – Transoesophageal echocardiogram
TSH – Thyroid stimulating hormone
TTE – Trans-thoracic echocardiogram

VLDL – Very low density lipoprotein
VMA – Vanillylmandelic acid
VPBs – Ventricular premature beats
VSD – Ventricular septal defect
VT – Ventricular tachycardia

WCC – White cell count

1 This was obtained from a 42-year-old man from Turkey with a 3-month history of fatigue, abdominal distension and breathlessness.
i. What is the diagnosis?
ii. Give three possible causes.
iii. What physical signs are characteristically observed in this disorder?

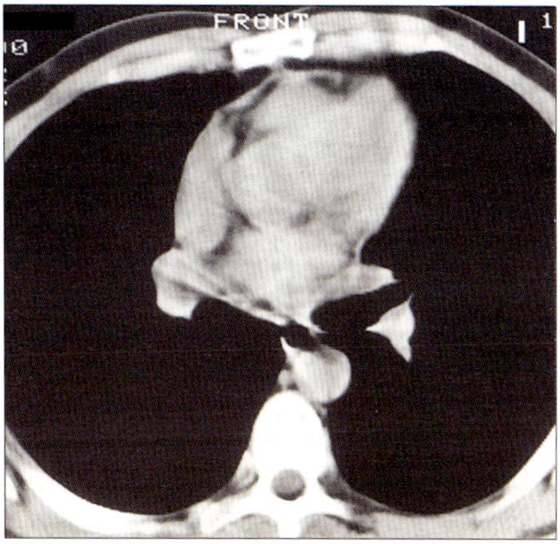

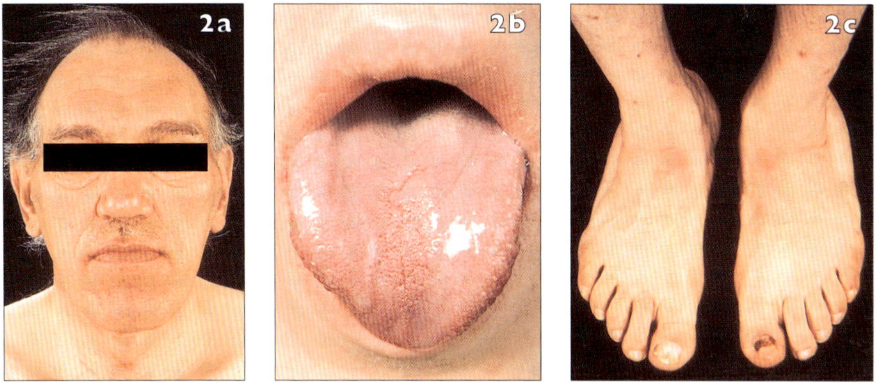

2 This 50-year-old man complained of angina of effort. On examination he was found to have a blood pressure of 160/100 mmHg.
i. Suggest a reason for the high blood pressure.
ii. Suggest a reason for the angina.
iii. What is the underlying condition and what effect would definitive treatment have on the cardiovascular symptoms?

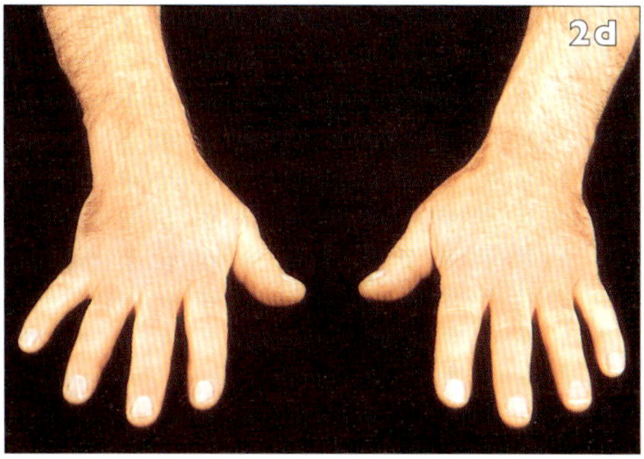

1 i. The computed tomography (CT) scan shows calcification of the pericardium, but the heart is not enlarged. (*NB* If the calcification had developed in the thrombus lining an aneurysm or infarction scar, the calcium would not be on the outside of the cardiac outline, but would be limited to the thrombus lining the area of thinned and bulging wall.) The clinical history gives a hint as to the possibility of a tuberculous origin of the disease. The other clinical features described are typical of cardiac constriction, as well as the non-specific symptoms, e.g. fatigue, which are common in this condition.
ii. Possible causes of constrictive pericarditis include tuberculosis, previous pyogenic infection, and rheumatoid arthritis. Constriction occurs rarely after cardiac surgery and in uraemia, but most cases are idiopathic. Besides CT scanning, as shown, magnetic resonance imaging (MRI) can also be of value.
iii. Typical physical signs are those of right ventricular failure. There are prominent x and y descents in the jugular venous pressure (JVP); this is so even in atrial fibrillation. Kussmaul's sign (a rise in JVP with inspiration) may or may not be present. Ankle oedema, hepatosplenomegaly and ascites are common. An early third heart sound (S3) may be heard (incorrectly known as a pericardial knock). Atrial fibrillation is common and pulsus paradoxus occurs in about 50% of cases. (*NB* In cardiac tamponade, the y descent is absent.)

2 i. 2a shows an acromegalic facies; also shown are the patient's tongue (**2b**), feet (**2c**), and hands (**2d**). The underlying diagnosis is acromegaly. Hypertension is very prevalent (20–50%) in acromegaly and may be caused by arterial smooth muscle hypertrophy due to the excess of growth hormone with or without increased total body sodium and increased plasma volume.
ii. The combination of impaired glucose tolerance (often to the point of frank diabetes) and hypertension markedly promote coronary artery disease in acromegalics.
iii. The definitive treatment is either surgery or radiotherapy, although bromocriptine will produce tumour shrinkage. However, despite these measures, blood pressure often remains elevated. The arterial disease and ventricular hypertrophy which develop in acromegaly do not regress.

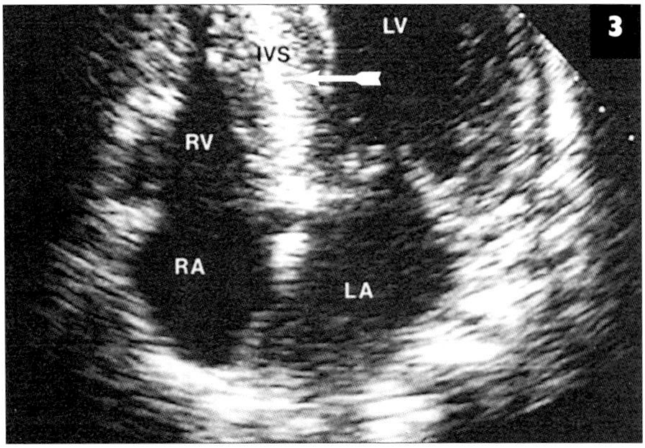

3 **i.** What is the major structure arrowed?
ii. What abnormality is shown?
iii. Is this specific to any particular condition or group of conditions?

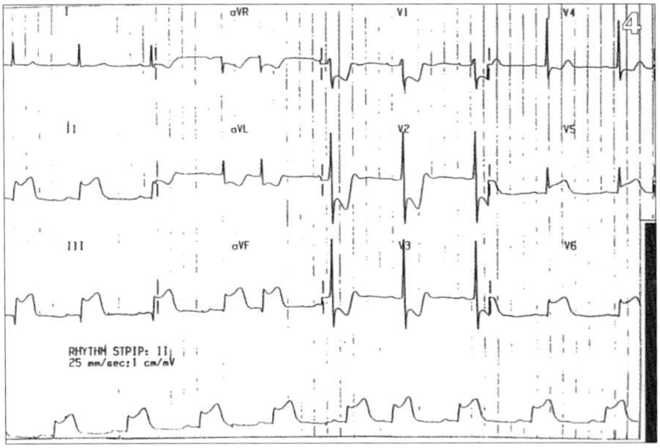

4 A 63-year-old man was admitted to a coronary care unit (CCU) with a 2-hour history of chest pain. Physical examination on arrival was essentially normal. Following an electrocardiogram (ECG), shown here, he received urgent thrombolysis, 2 hours after which he became hypotensive with a systolic blood pressure of 80 mmHg. His heart rate was 110/min and regular, JVP was elevated above the sternal angle, and heart sounds were normal. Peripheral pulses were symmetrically and equally palpable, the chest was clear, and abdominal examination was normal.
Investigations show:
Full blood count (FBC): haemoglobin (Hb), 15.2 g/dl; white cell count (WCC), 15 x 10^9/l; platelets, 388 x 10^9/l.
U&E: sodium, 136 mmol/l; potassium, 5.1 mmol/l; urea, 9 mmol/l (BUN, 25 mg/dl); creatinine, 90 µmol/l (1.1 mg/dl).
Chest radiograph: normal sized heart, mediastinal width normal, lung fields clear.
i. What is the original diagnosis (see ECG)?
ii. What is the cause of hypotension in this case?
iii. List two non-invasive tests which could be performed on the CCU to confirm the diagnosis.

3 **i.** The structure arrowed is the ventricular septum.
ii. There is gross and asymmetric hypertrophy of the septum, with normal thickness of the posterior ventricular wall. The left ventricular chamber dimensions are reduced.
iii. Although hypertrophy of the ventricular septum is a sensitive marker of hypertrophic cardiomyopathy [HCM, sometimes known as idiopathic hypertrophic subaortic stenosis (IHSS)], a disorder characterised by myocardial hypertrophy without any apparent external cause, it is not specific. A ratio of ventricular septal thickness:left ventricular posterior wall thickness of >1.5 is very suggestive of HCM, but septal hypertrophy is also found in other conditions which produce left ventricular hypertrophy, such as valvar and subvalvar aortic stenosis and essential hypertension. In addition, septal thickness increases relatively and absolutely with age. [It is also possible for a patient to have hypertrophic cardiomyopathy with normal echocardiographic appearance of the septum. Some populations (e.g. in Japan) have a high prevalence of apical hypertrophy and, rarely, hypertrophy is largely confined to the right ventricle (in the absence of any secondary cause of right ventricular hypertrophy).]

4 **i.** The diagnosis is inferolateral myocardial infarction with posterior extension. There is ST segment elevation in leads II, III, and aVf, V5 and V6, consistent with acute inferolateral myocardial infarction. The R waves in V1–V3 are dominant and the ST segments are significantly depressed in these leads. These changes are reciprocal to the changes seen in myocardial infarction in the anterior wall and are suggestive of posterior wall infarction. Inferior myocardial infarction is often associated with posterior wall infarction because the same artery supplies both these territories. Right coronary artery occlusion is usually implicated; however, the same ECG changes can occur with circumflex artery occlusion when it is dominant and provides the posterior descending artery (see also **176**).
ii. The most likely cause of hypotension is right ventricular infarction. The differential diagnosis comprises pulmonary embolism or an acute ventricular septal defect (VSD), but it is too early for either. The usual timing for thromboembolism is approximately 72 hours. VSD is a recognised complication of anterior or inferior myocardial infarction and is characterised by similar signs to those seen in this patient; however, in acute VSD there is a new pan-systolic murmur and the chest radiograph often reveals an enlarged heart and pulmonary oedema. An allergic reaction to streptokinase could cause profound hypotension, but this usually occurs within 30 minutes of commencing the drug.
iii. Two non-invasive tests which could be performed on the CCU include a right-sided ECG, which may reveal ST segment elevation in V4R, and an echocardiogram to demonstrate a dilated and hypokinetic right ventricle.

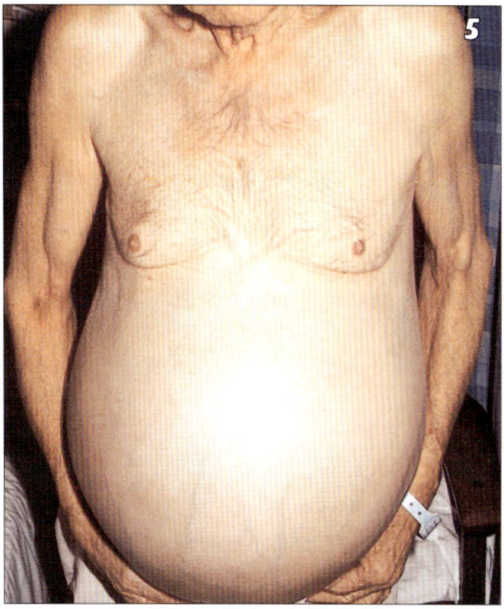

5 This 60-year-old former miner used to be a heavy smoker. He gave up 3 years previously. He has become increasingly breathless, to the extent that he cannot move more than about 10 m before being out of breath. He has been treated so far with digoxin and diuretics only.
i. What can you see?
ii. What do you expect his plasma renin and total body sodium levels to be?

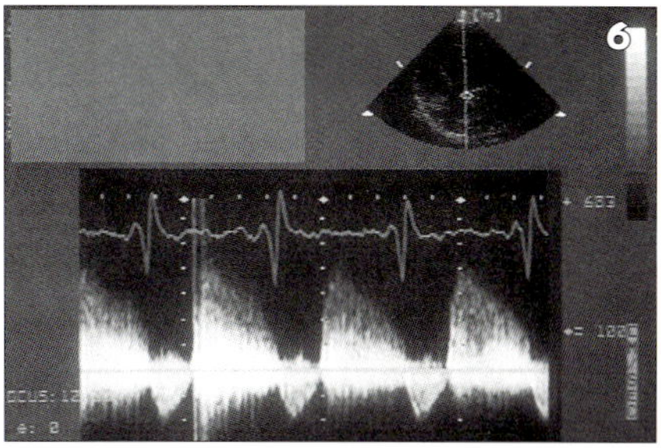

6 **i.** What is this investigation?
ii. What is the diagnosis?
iii. Estimate the severity of the problem.

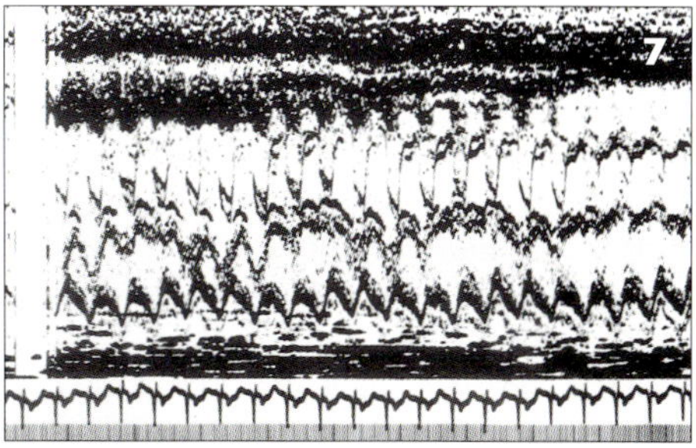

7 A cardiological opinion was sought urgently regarding a 32-year-old man who was being investigated for non-specific ill-health and vague chest pains. His blood pressure had fallen to 80/50 mmHg over the course of 3 hours, his pulse had risen to 130 b.p.m., with pulsus paradoxus and a rise in venous pressure. The investigation shown was performed prior to an emergency procedure.
i. What is the investigation and what does it show?
ii. What is the diagnosis?
iii. What should be done?

5 **i.** This man has biventricular failure. He developed pulmonary disease due to a combination of smoking and dust exposure in the course of his work. He also has ischaemic heart disease. A manifestation of the right heart failure is the distension of the abdomen with ascites.
ii. In congestive cardiac failure, the response of the kidney is physiologically similar to that in hypovolaemia. In the face of a reduction in cardiac output, salt and water are retained in order to restore the arterial blood volume. This is mediated, at least in part, by the increase in renin secretion evoked by the drop in arterial pressure registered in the afferent renal tubule. The rise in renin leads to an increase in aldosterone secretion and, in turn, to an increase in sodium resorption and retention with concomitant water retention. Thus, both plasma renin and total body sodium are increased.

6 **i.** This is an echocardiographic study in continuous-wave Doppler mode.
ii. The diagnosis is aortic regurgitation.
iii. The Doppler technique is semi-quantitative rather than accurately quantitative in the case of regurgitant valve disease. One index of the severity of the valvar regurgitation is the rate of decrease in velocity of the jet of regurgitant blood into the left ventricle. In the example shown, the steep slope indicates that there is a rapid reduction in the gradient between the aorta and left ventricle and therefore the regurgitation is severe. Perhaps a more precise measure using echocardiography would be a comparison between aortic flow and either trans-mitral or trans-pulmonic flow.

7 **i.** The investigation is an M mode echocardiogram. It shows tachycardia, a pericardial effusion located both anteriorly and posteriorly, and collapse of the right atrial and right ventricular free wall during diastole. The latter is an important early sign which may be found even before haemodynamic compromise.
ii. The history (consistent with pericarditis) and physical signs (tachycardia, hypotension, and pulsus paradoxus) point strongly to a diagnosis of pericardial tamponade, even without the echocardiogram. The last is of value in documenting the presence and size of the pericardial effusion, since in the absence of the latter the diagnosis of tamponade is extremely unlikely, unless post-cardiac surgical thrombus or loculated fluid is compressing the heart. In fact, demonstration of the echocardiographic signs listed in **i.** above, especially the right ventricular diastolic collapse, and an increase in the right ventricular dimension during inspiration put the diagnosis beyond doubt.
iii. With haemodynamic and echocardiographic monitoring and intravenous fluid support, percutaneous pericardiocentesis should be performed without delay. Ideally, it should be done in the cardiac catheterisation laboratory.

8 This chest radiograph was taken from a 22-year-old intravenous drug abuser who presented with pleuritic chest pain, fever, and a non-productive cough. What is the abnormality?

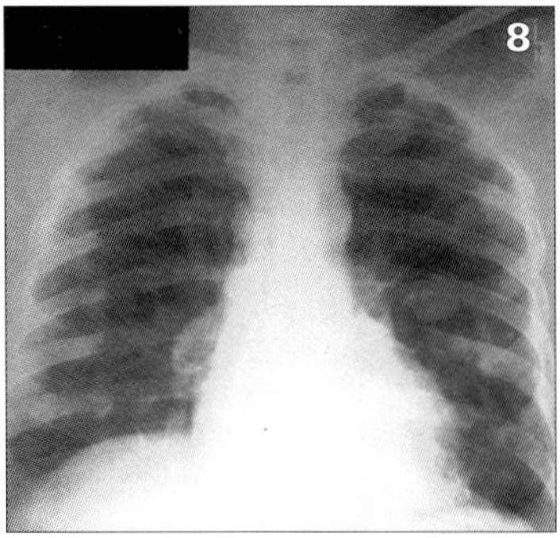

9 This is a 2D echocardiogram of a 24-year-old man who presented with breathlessness, sharp left sided inframammary pain, and palpitations. What is the diagnosis?

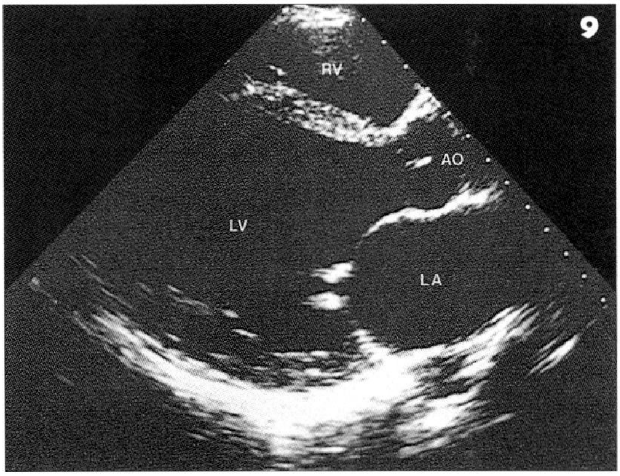

10 A 54-year-old waitress complained of chest pain on exertion. Her past history and physical examination were unremarkable. She developed this ECG appearance on exercise testing. An echocardiogram was normal, as was coronary arteriography.

i. What does the ECG show?
ii. What is the working diagnosis?
iii. What is the prognosis?

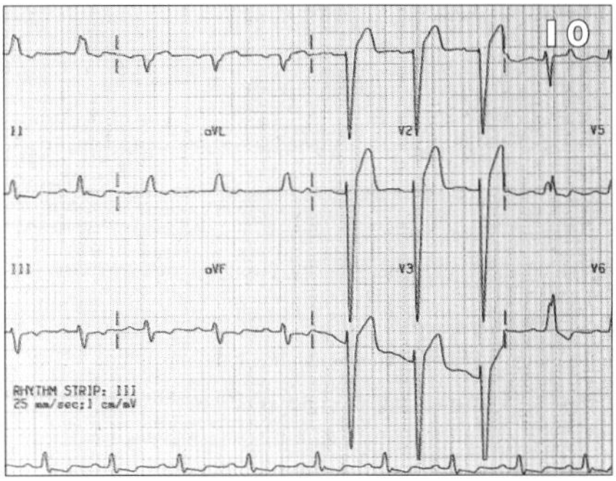

8 The radiograph demonstrates multiple cavitating lesions. These almost certainly represent infected emboli from right-sided infective endocarditis, which is common in intravenous drug abusers. A murmur is not always audible in tricuspid endocarditis. The bacterial agent most commonly implicated is *Staphylococcus aureus*. Fungal endocarditis also occurs with increased frequency in such patients.

9 The echocardiogram demonstrates an enlarged left atrium and a dilated left ventricle, with ventricular walls of normal thickness. The most likely cause of this appearance in such a young patient is viral myocarditis, resulting in a cardiomyopathy. The most common cause of viral myocarditis is the Coxsackie B virus group. One-third of patients give a clear history of a recent viral illness. The majority of patients present with fatigue, breathlessness, palpitation and chest pain, characteristic of pericarditis. Atrial fibrillation and ventricular ectopics are common, but ventricular tachycardia and degrees of atrioventricular block may occur. In a few patients, viral myocarditis may manifest as cardiogenic shock. The physical signs are those of cardiac failure. Auscultation often reveals a third heart sound and murmurs of both mitral and tricuspid regurgitation.

An ECG usually demonstrates non-specific ST segment and T wave changes, although tachyarrhythmias, heart block and bundle branch block may be noted.

A chest radiograph shows variable degrees of cardiomegaly and pulmonary oedema. Echocardiography is essential to document ventricular size and function, and an associated pericardial effusion. The quantification of functional valve regurgitation is achieved by means of Doppler echocardiography. Infiltrative cardiac muscle disorders, which can present in a similar fashion, can also be excluded using echocardiography. Cardiac catheterisation is necessary to exclude coronary artery disease. Cardiac biopsy is only positive for viral myocarditis in 5–6% of patients with this clinical diagnosis, so there is a disparity between clinical and biopsy findings. Moreover, various immunosuppressive treatment regimes have not altered the prognosis when compared with patients receiving treatment for heart failure alone. Routine cardiac biopsy is not necessary in making the diagnosis of viral myocarditis.

10 **i.** The ECG shows left bundle branch block (LBBB) – note the increased QRS complex duration, the absence of septal q waves in V5 and V6, I, and aVL, and the absence of an R´ or r´ in V1 (which would indicate the presence of right bundle branch block). In LBBB, depolarisation of the interventricular septum occurs in the opposite direction from normal, i.e. from right to left. Since septal depolarisation is the first part of the entire left ventricular depolarisation process and therefore electrocardiographically constitutes the earliest part of the QRS complex, the normal 'septal' q in V5 and V6 disappears.

ii. In this woman with chest pain on exertion, LBBB developed, despite there being smooth normal coronary arteries at angiography. She is not a case of syndrome X in the widely accepted use of the term, but might have an early cardiomyopathy and an isolated fascicular block.

11 **i.** What is shown here?
ii. What is the diagnosis and why are the toes blue?

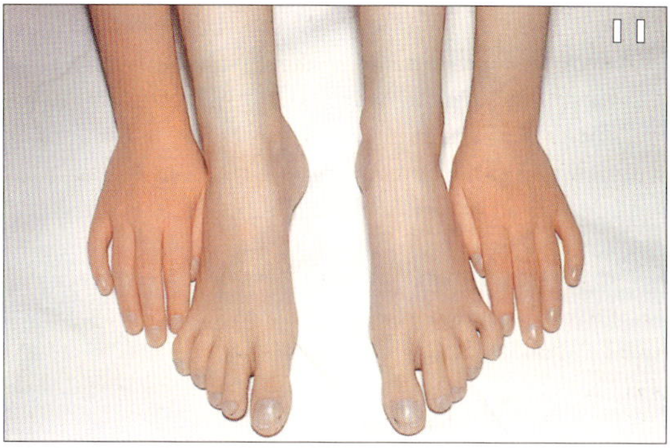

12 This is an M mode echocardiogram.
i. What are the abnormalities?
ii. What is the diagnosis?
(RV, right ventricle; LV, left ventricle; AML, anterior mitral valve leaflet; PML, posterior mitral valve leaflet; END, endocardium.)

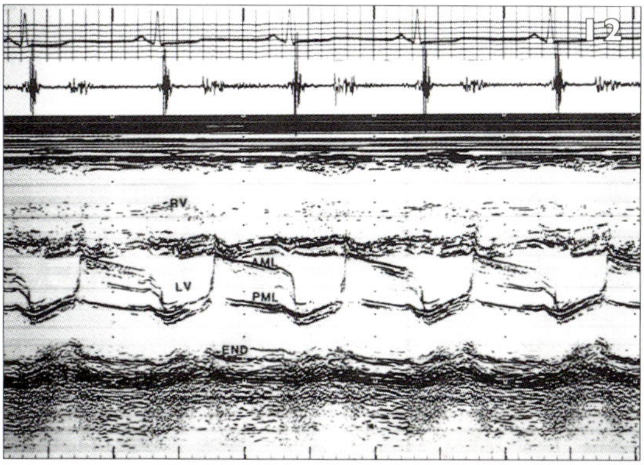

13 A 30-year-old woman from Eastern Europe was admitted on the general medical take, having presented with fever, breathlessness and tachycardia and with a presumptive diagnosis of atypical pneumonia. The admitting physician observed non-specific ST segment changes and a PR interval of 280 ms on the ECG. A few hours later he also noticed the skin lesions shown here.
i. What can you see?
ii. What is the underlying diagnosis?
iii. How would you manage this case?

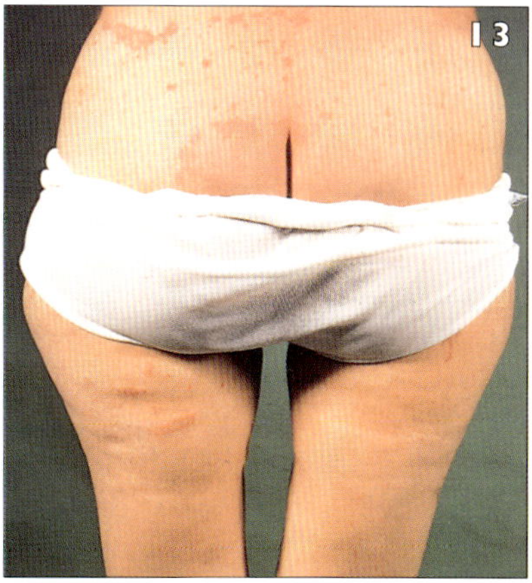

11 i. Shown is clubbing of the toes, but not of the fingers. This is due to differential cyanosis between the feet and hands (see below).
ii. The underlying disorder is patency of the arterial duct (PDA) with shunt reversal. This occurs as an isolated lesion in 1 in 1500 live births, where it takes the form of a wide and smooth conduit which permits communication (and also therefore shunting) between the systemic and pulmonary circulations. If there is free flow with pulmonary hypertension, shunt reversal can occur due to a rise in pulmonary vascular resistance. Deoxygenated blood is returned to the systemic circulation below the level of origin of the subclavian arteries. Thus, cyanosis affects the lower but not the upper limbs; therefore the toes are clubbed and blue, but not the fingers.

12 i. The three abnormalities are: (a) thickening of the anterior mitral valve leaflet, such that the classic M-shaped pattern of the anterior leaflet is lost; (b) mitral valve excursion is reduced; and (c) anterior motion of the posterior mitral valve leaflet in diastole.
ii. These abnormalities are characteristic of rheumatic mitral valve disease.

13 i. and **ii.** Erythema marginatum is present – essentially a pinkish rash with raised edges and a white centre, which is a transient phenomenon in about 20% of cases of acute rheumatic fever. The rings or crescent shapes and location on the trunk of this subject are characteristic. Again, the history gives many clues as to the underlying disorder. Acute rheumatic fever is now rare in the West, but still a relatively common affliction of young people in Eastern Europe, Asia, Africa, and South America. In a woman of 30, this would not be a first attack and she would probably have pre-existing valve disease. Rheumatic fever is probably due to an autoimmune reaction to a preceding streptococcal throat or skin infection. Presentation may be with obvious cardiological symptoms which indicate an underlying carditis, e.g. new or altered heart murmurs, cardiomegaly or heart failure, pericardial effusion, or ECG changes of pericarditis, myocarditis, atrioventricular block, or other arrhythmias. These, along with polyarthritis, chorea, erythema marginatum, and subcutaneous nodules, constitute the major Duckett Jones diagnostic criteria. The minor criteria include fever, joint pains, raised erythrocyte sedimentation rate (ESR), previous rheumatic fever and PR interval prolongation. This woman had two major criteria, adequate for a firm diagnosis.
iii. The aims of treatment in acute rheumatic fever are relief of symptoms and limitation of damage to the heart. Bed rest is necessary and penicillin should be given to eradicate streptococcal infection. Salicylates (with steroids if necessary) ameliorate symptoms, but probably do not affect the progression of valvar damage. Prophylaxis with penicillin should be continued long term – i.e. for 5 years).

14 A 58-year-old woman presented to the emergency department with severe dyspnoea. She was taken urgently to the cardiac catheter laboratory.
i. What is the diagnosis?
ii. What treatment should be administered?

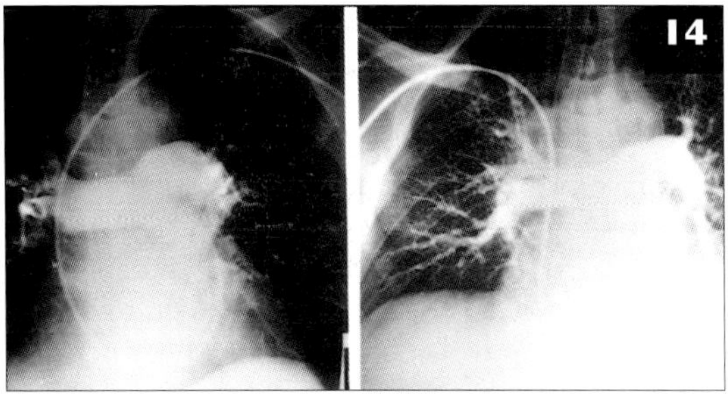

15 **i.** What is shown in these radiographs?
ii. What is the diagnosis?

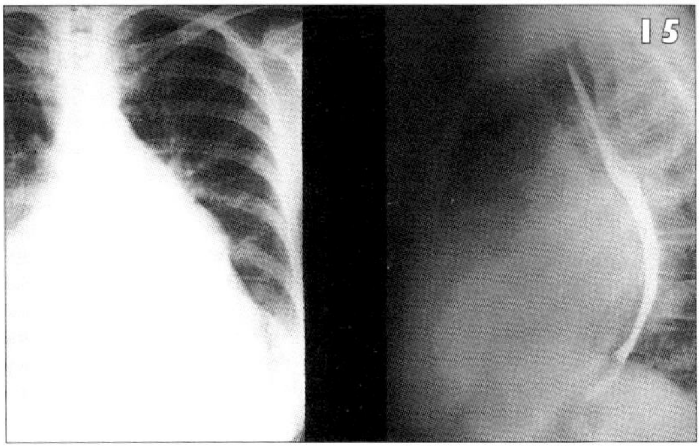

16 A 53-year-old man was admitted with a 12-hour history of central chest pain. Physical examination was normal and an ECG was obtained (shown here). He was treated immediately and observed on the CCU, but after 24 hours he became very breathless. On examination he was clammy, his heart rate was 135/minute, systolic blood pressure was 70 mmHg, and JVP was elevated to the ear lobes. Widespread lung crackles were heard and on cardiac auscultation there was a loud pan-systolic murmur and thrill internal to the apex.

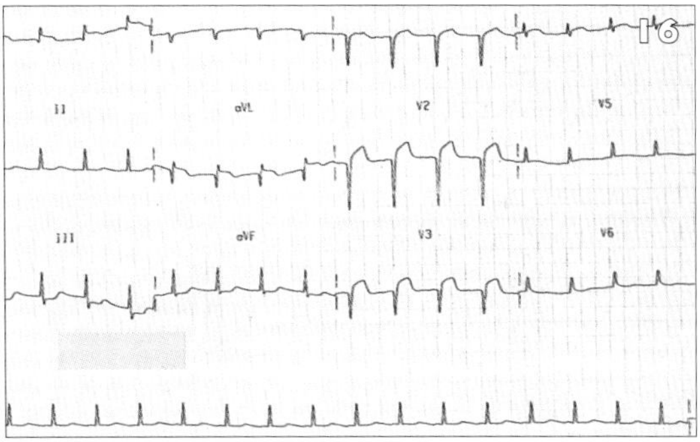

i. What is the ECG diagnosis?
ii. Which complication has occurred?
iii. How would you confirm your diagnosis?
iv. What is the management?

14 i. This angiogram shows a segmental pulmonary artery occlusion. It was obtained during the further investigation and management of the woman's acute pulmonary embolism.
ii. There are both general and specific considerations in the management of acute pulmonary embolism. Resuscitation should be commenced with fluids, oxygen, and head-down tilt (if necessary). Diuretics and vasodilators are harmful. Heparin is administered as an intravenous bolus of 15,000 IU (215 IU/kg) followed by about 500 IU/kg/day. Heparin's principle role is probably the prevention of further thromboembolism, while the body's intrinsic thrombolytic mechanisms deal with the clot which has already formed. In severe cases, thrombolytic therapy (usually streptokinase, 250,000–500,000 IU loading dose over half-an-hour followed by 100,000 IU/hour) can be administered, often via cardiac catheterisation if, as in the case shown, this has been used to confirm the diagnosis acutely. The thrombotic material visualised at angiography should be pushed further down the pulmonary artery to free the proximal branches by fragmenting it and streptokinase infused locally These measures will unload the right ventricle. Subsequently, conventional therapy with anticoagulants is indicated.

15 i. The radiographs reveal calcification of the mitral valve and enlargement of the left atrium, left ventricle, right atrium and ventricle, and pulmonary artery. Kerley B lines and small pleural effusions can also be seen, with upper lobe diversion of the pulmonary venous blood.
ii. The underlying diagnosis is post rheumatic mixed mitral valve disease. The calcified mitral valve has been moderately stenotic for years; in addition, the immobility of the valve leaflets has rendered the valve regurgitant. Hence in addition to the left atrial enlargement which might be a feature of mitral stenosis alone, the left ventricular enlargement is the clue to the mitral regurgitation. As the pulmonary pressures have risen, right ventricular dilatation, tricuspid regurgitation and right atrial enlargement have occurred. The Kerley B lines, upper lobe blood diversion and small pleural effusions are indicative of left ventricular failure.

16. i. Anterior myocardial infarction.
ii. VSD, which can occur with inferior or anterior infarction, but is more common with the latter. It presents with haemodynamic compromise and a pan-systolic murmur.
iii. The diagnosis is best confirmed by echocardiography with colour flow Doppler, which immediately identifies the problem and shows left and right ventricular function. The differential diagnosis in a patient with sudden haemodynamic compromise and a new murmur after myocardial infarction is either VSD or acute mitral regurgitation following papillary muscle rupture. (See also **130**.)
iv. Early surgery is recommended. The condition carries a high mortality if treatment is delayed. Intra-aortic balloon pumping is of particular help pre-operatively in reducing the shunt, lowering the left atrial pressure, and improving forward flow, but operation should not be delayed.

17 This 35-year-old man collapsed without warning on three occasions in 4 months. There were no premonitory symptoms. Give a likely explanation and suggest the most effective treatment.

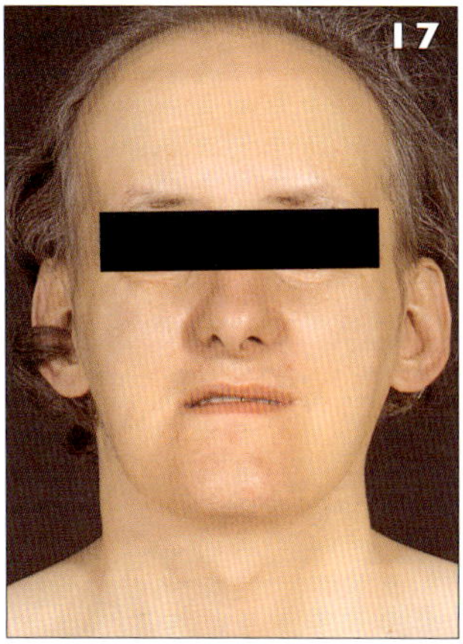

18 A 47-year-old woman with sore legs and a year-long history of breathlessness on exertion gave the chest radiograph shown. She complained of occasional palpitations and a specialist cardiological consultation was arranged. She died suddenly, prior to being seen. Suggest an underlying diagnosis and account for the clinical course.

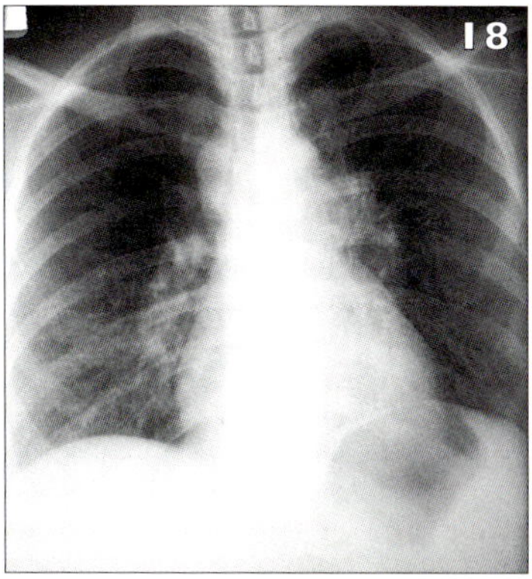

19 A 34-year-old black woman had complained of being very breathless as she approached term with her fifth pregnancy. She was admitted at 36 weeks with a blood pressure of 140/85 mmHg and labour was induced. However, within days the woman developed worsening cardiac failure and died. The specimen shown was obtained at autopsy. What is the diagnosis and what is the cause?

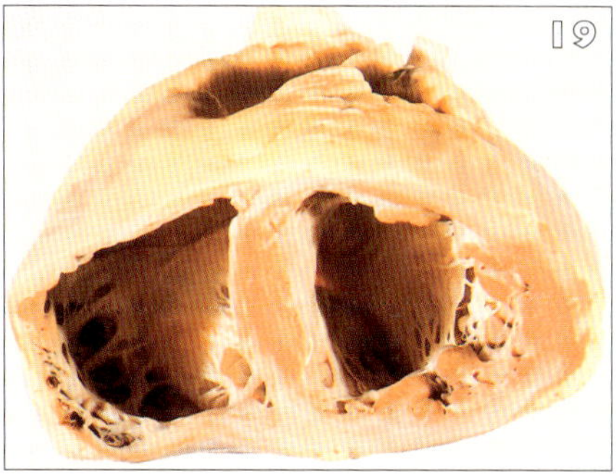

17 The myopathic facies, frontal balding, wasting of the facial muscles, and ptosis suggest a diagnosis of dystrophia myotonica. Among the neuromuscular diseases, dystrophia myotonica is relatively common. It has an incidence of 3–5 per 100,000 and is inherited as an autosomal dominant disorder, due to a deficit on chromosome 19. Weakness of the neck flexors is typical, with atrophy of the sternomastoids. Myotonia can be shown as a delay in relaxation of skeletal muscle after mechanical or electrical stimulation. Other associated features are cataracts, premature baldness, testicular atrophy, and dysfunction of visceral smooth muscle, such as the gut or uterus. With respect to the cardiovascular system, it is the cardiac conducting tissues which are affected principally; fatty infiltration, fibrosis and atrophy of the sinoatrial node, atrioventricular node, bundle of His and bundle branches have all been found post-mortem. Myocardial dystrophy may manifest itself as a mild cardiomyopathy, but leads to heart failure in less than 10% of cases (cf. Friedreich's ataxia). The most common electrocardiographic abnormalities are prolongation of the PR interval, left axis deviation, prolongation of the QRS complex, and right bundle branch block. His–Purkinje disease can progress rapidly to complete heart block, producing Stokes–Adams attacks, as here. Permanent pacing provides effective treatment.

18 The chest radiograph shows hilar lymphadenopathy and fibrosis. The woman had sarcoidosis, with erythema nodosum causing the leg lesions. In this case there was considerable cardiac involvement, with myocardial infiltration provoking ventricular arrhythmias which were ultimately fatal.

Sarcoidosis is a granulomatous disorder characterised by the presence within organs of the body of epithelioid tubercles (without the caseation which distinguishes tuberculosis). Cardiac involvement in sarcoidosis is infrequent, about 1.5%, but the incidence is higher in patients who die of the underlying disease. The myocardium (especially the left ventricular free wall, ventricular septum, and papillary muscles) has numerous areas replaced by granulomatous tissue. There is often extensive fibrosis, which often involves the conducting tissues. The fibrosis causes a stiffening of the left ventricle with impairment of left ventricular diastolic function, resulting in a restrictive or congestive cardiomyopathy. Heart block and arrhythmias are frequent and sudden cardiac death is a common end.

19 The post-mortem specimen is of a globally dilated heart. In the context of the clinical history this is a typical case of peripartum cardiomyopathy, an uncommon disorder with an incidence of about 1 in 3000 pregnancies. Biopsy specimens from hearts with peripartum cardiomyopathy usually show acute myocarditis. As in cases of myocarditis outside of pregnancy, the disease can be rapidly fatal, as here. However, if it is not, considerable improvement can occur. It is unusual for any evidence of viral infection to be found. The myocardial inflammation may be immunologically mediated with the fetus as antigen.

20 A 54-year-old woman was investigated for increasing breathlessness. She had been noted to have had a murmur 20 years previously. Cardiac catheterisation results were as follows:

Chamber	*Pressure (mmHg)*	*O_2 saturation (%)*
RA	8 (mean)	66%
RV	42/3	66%
PA	44/18	67%
PCWP	25 (mean)	–
LV	120/3	95%
Aorta	128/70	95%

(RA, right atrium; RV, right ventricle; PA, pulmonary artery; PCWP, pulmonary capillary wedge pressure; LV, left ventricle.)
i. List three abnormalities.
ii. What is the diagnosis?

21 A 58-year-old man had a prolonged (>1 h) episode of chest pain associated with profuse sweating, nausea, and vomiting. He was told that he had suffered a heart attack. After a difficult first week, the patient's course was reasonable over the following 4 months, although his effort tolerance was significantly curtailed.

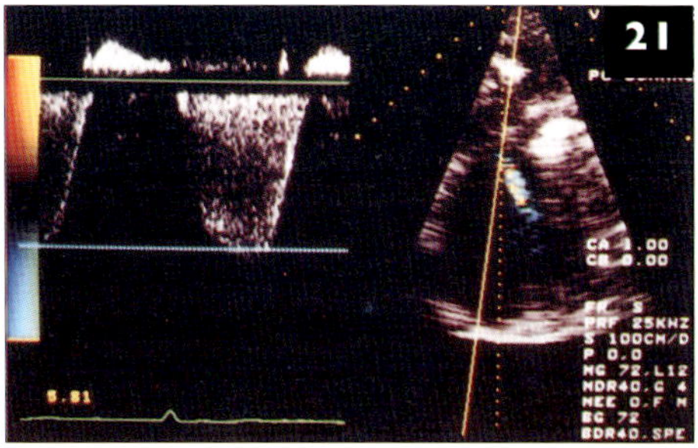

i. The transducer in this investigation was placed in a low parasternal position. What structure is being assessed?
ii. What does the investigation show?
iii. What earlier event do you think caused the problem demonstrated?

22 This scan was obtained from a 3-year-old boy whose only symptom was a moderate reduction in effort tolerance.
i. What is the abnormality shown?
ii. What are the strengths and weaknesses of this technology in the investigation of the type of abnormality shown?

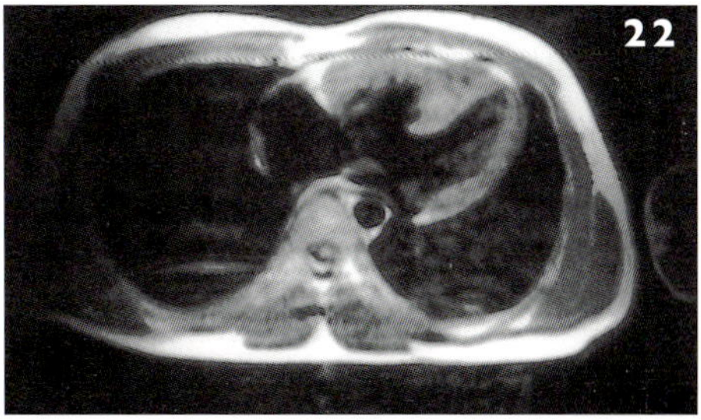

20 **i.** Three abnormalities are (a) raised right atrial, right ventricular, and pulmonary artery pressures, suggesting pulmonary hypertension; (b) elevated pulmonary capillary wedge pressure, indicative of raised left atrial pressure; and (c) a gradient of 27 mmHg across the mitral valve in diastole (for normal ranges see Appendix).
ii. The findings are consistent with severe mitral stenosis and secondary pulmonary hypertension.

21 **i.** The echo view is a parasternal long-axis view of the tricuspid valve.
ii. This is a continuous-wave Doppler study which reveals significant tricuspid regurgitation.
iii. The clinical history here describes features suggestive of an acute inferior myocardial infarction with extensive right ventricular involvement. The right ventricular infarction produced right ventricular dysfunction, with associated functional incompetence of the tricuspid valve. Generally, 2D echocardiography in functional tricuspid regurgitation reveals only the non-specific effects of right ventricular volume overload associated with tricuspid regurgitation of any cause, e.g. right ventricular dilatation and reversed septal motion. Doppler echocardiography is a very sensitive technique for detecting even the mild degrees of tricuspid regurgitation present in normal individuals. An estimate of the severity may be made according to the distance back into the right atrium that the regurgitant jet reaches. In the presence of tricuspid regurgitation, right ventricular systolic pressure can be obtained from the velocity (V) of the regurgitant jet, in that the systolic transvalvar pressure gradient is approximately $4V^2$. The right ventricular systolic pressure is then approximately equal to ($4V^2$ + right atrial pressure). JVP can be used as an approximation to the right atrial pressure.

22 **i.** This MRI scan shows a ventricular septal defect.
ii. This is a gated spin echo image with magnetic resonance. The method is particularly good for the demonstration of atrial and ventricular septal defects, as well as abnormalities of the inlets, outlets, and connections of the cardiac chambers. In general, a 3D acquisition is performed in the form of multiple slices, typically of 10 mm thickness, in three orthogonal planes. If necessary, a second acquisition can be made, offset a few millimetres from the first. High field strengths, e.g. 1.5 T, are necessary to produce images of adequate clarity. The image acquisition process is quite slow, e.g. about 3 minutes per data set, so the method is unsuitable for young children. Functional data, such as the detection of areas of turbulence, can be obtained by means of gradient echo sequences with long echo times. Short echo times permit flow velocity mapping, allowing the measurement of absolute flow; pressure gradients can be obtained in a fashion analogous to that for Doppler echocardiography and the degree of ventricular shunting can be calculated. This is largely a research technique, since the same information can be gained much more simply and less expensively by echocardiography.

23 The phonocardiogram (**23a**) was obtained from a young woman said to have a 'hole in the heart'. The patient's ECG is also shown (**23b**).

i. What abnormality can be seen in the patient's phonocardiogram?

ii. What does the ECG show?

iii. What do you think the 'hole in the heart' might be?

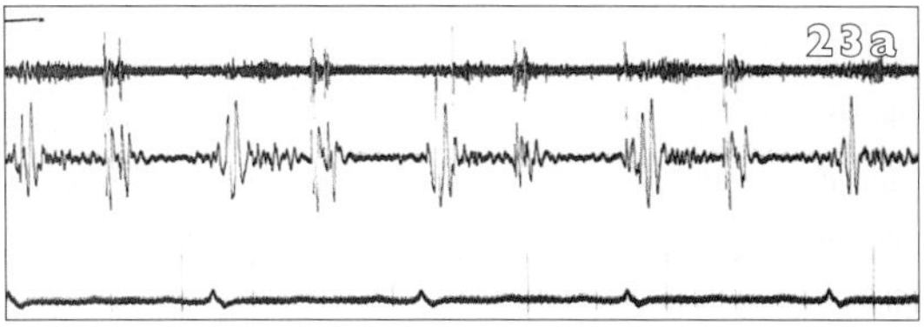

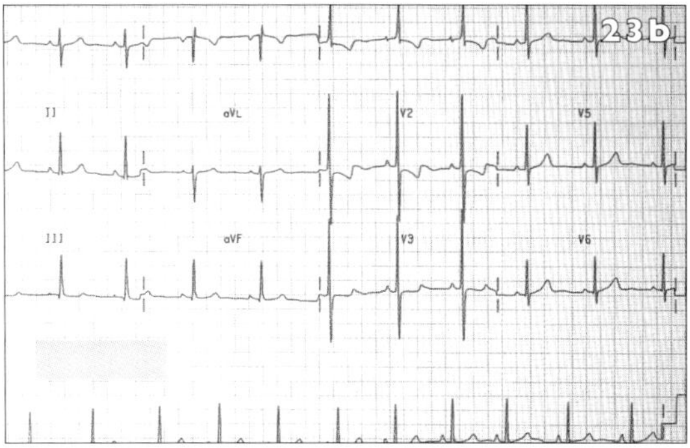

24 These two images (**24a**, **24b**) were obtained at angiography in the same patient, a 65-year-old woman who experiences moderate angina of effort. She has a normal resting ECG and inferolateral ischaemia on exercise, but good ventricular function.

i. What is the diagnosis?

ii. What are the options for intervention?

iii. What is the evidence to favour one interventional option over the other in these circumstances?

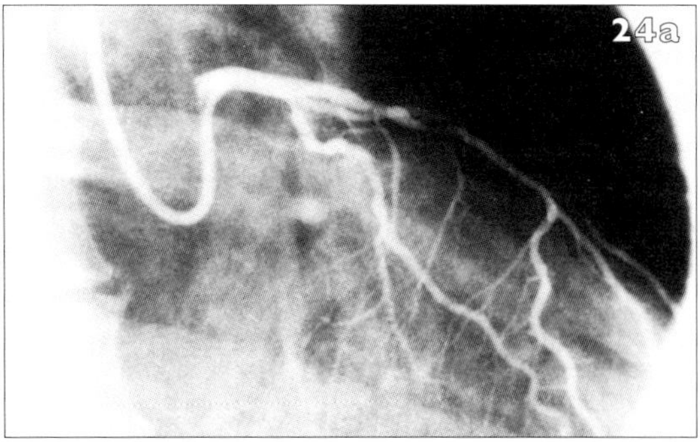

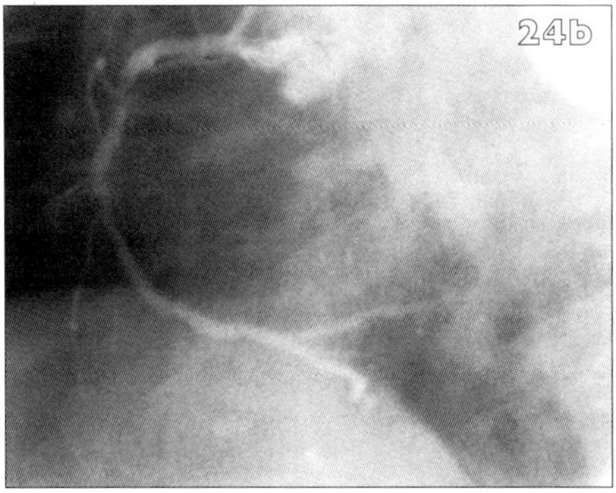

23 **i.** The phonocardiogram of this patient shows a soft ejection systolic murmur, best heard in the pulmonary area, and a prolonged time interval between the aortic and pulmonary components of the second heart sound (i.e. widely split A2 and P2). These signs are suggestive of an atrial septal defect (ASD). The systolic murmur is soft and related to increased forward flow; there is no murmur of mitral regurgitation.
ii. The ECG shows right axis deviation and right ventricular hypertrophy (note the tall R waves in V1–V3 and T wave inversion in V1 and V2).
iii. The combination of phonocardiographic evidence of ASD and right axis deviation makes the 'hole in the heart' likely to be an ostium secundum ASD. The right axis deviation and right ventricular hypertrophy are consistent with right ventricular cavity enlargement in secundum-type ASD. In contrast, ostium primum defects are associated with left axis deviation, presumably caused by the anterosuperior division of the left bundle branch being involved in the endocardial cushion defect, which is central to the aetiology of ostium primum ASD.

24 **i.** This woman has critical coronary artery stenoses affecting the left anterior descending coronary artery (LAD) (**24a**) and the right coronary artery (**24b**). The circumflex has no significant stenosis.
ii. This particular clinical situation, i.e. moderate angina with two-vessel coronary artery disease, can be a difficult one in that there is no clear-cut optimal treatment strategy. Thus, the woman could be managed medically, with optimal anti-anginal treatment and aspirin. If the symptoms remain severe, then either percutaneous angioplasty of the coronary stenoses or coronary artery bypass grafting (CABG) could be performed. Exercise testing or stress echocardiography could help define the threshold for myocardial ischaemia.
iii. As yet there is no consensus as to which revascularisation approach is superior. Consequently, the patient's preference will be a major determinant, bearing in mind that although percutaneous transluminal coronary angioplasty is a more immediate and smaller scale procedure, there is an increased risk of recurrence of symptoms due to restenosis and of need for repeat angioplasty or CABG surgery.

25 A 40-year-old man had undergone surgery in his teens for an asymptomatic disorder. After regular follow-up (which included chest radiography) for a number of years, he had the investigation shown in **25a**.

i. What is the investigation and what does it show?

ii. What was the original lesion?

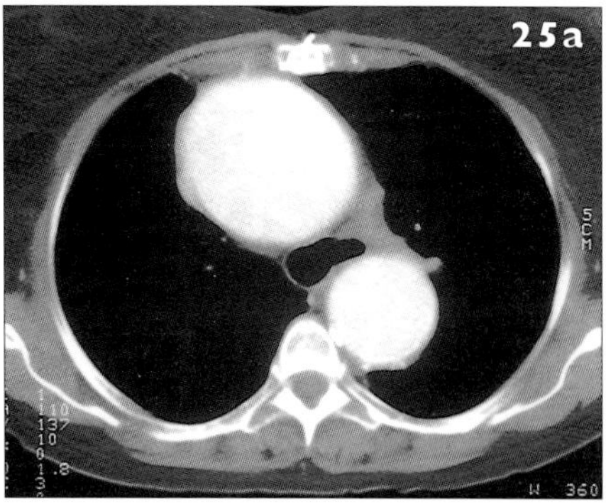

26 A 48-year-old man was investigated because of a recurrence of angina 18 months after an acute infarct. Where do you think the original infarct was?

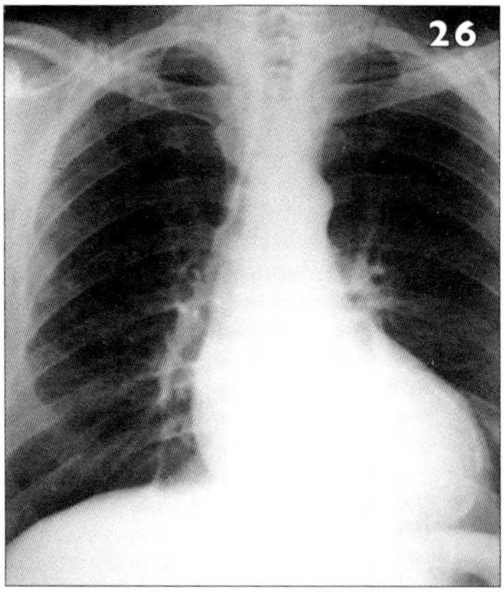

27 This was an incidental finding on a chest radiograph.

i. What is the visible abnormality?

ii. What are the causes of such an abnormality?

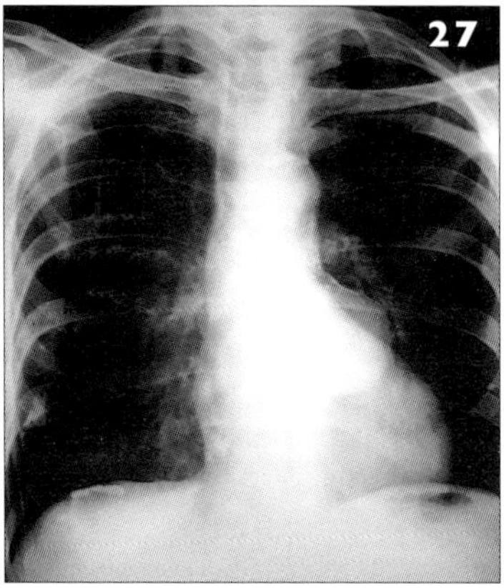

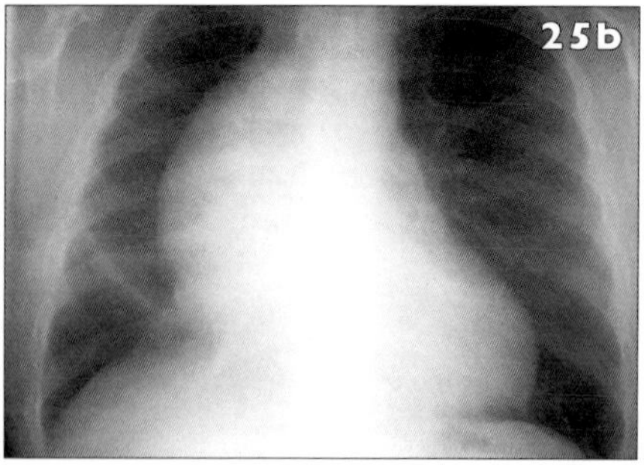

25 **i.** **25a** is an oblique MRI of the ascending aorta and aortic arch. It shows a posterior aneurysm at the site of a Dacron patch.
ii. This is a known complication of patch grafting. The asymptomatic patient had undergone resection of an uncomplicated coarctation of the aorta shortly after it was discovered about 20 years previously. A Dacron patch was used to replace the section of aorta resected. The man remained entirely asymptomatic for the next 20 years and the lesion shown was discovered on a chest radiograph (**25b**) during routine screening in the course of an assessment for life insurance. The MRI scan was performed during the further investigation of the patient prior to a decision regarding surgery for the resection of the aortic aneurysm at the site of the Dacron patch.

26 The chest radiograph shows calcification inside the cardiac apex. This is suggestive of an anteroapical site for the previous myocardial infarction.

27 **i.** The chest radiograph demonstrates an aneurysm of the descending aorta.
ii. Thoracic aortic aneurysms are uncommon. They are usually asymptomatic and identified on routine chest radiographs. The most common cause is arteriosclerosis. Cystic medial necrosis occurs in Marfan's syndrome and in Ehlers–Danlos syndrome. This can result in aortic dissection or rupture. In the past, syphilis caused thoracic aneurysms due to aortitis in the tertiary stage. The aortitis usually affected the ascending aorta and the aortic arch.

Thoracic aneurysms can become large and cause pressure symptoms. Large aneurysms are at risk of rupture, so surgical therapy is required to replace the aneurysm with a graft. The operation carries a high mortality and a large risk of paraplegia.

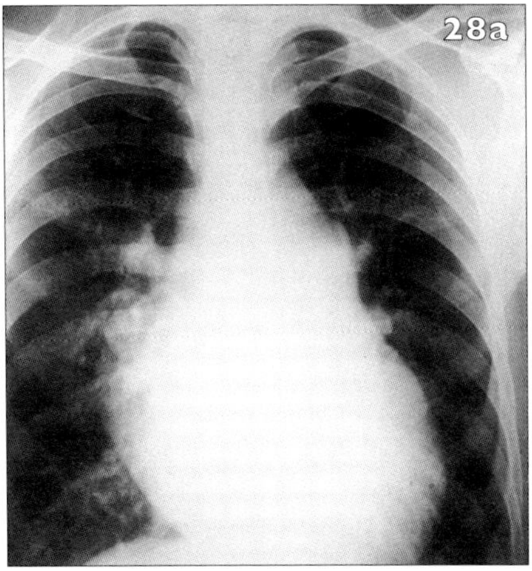

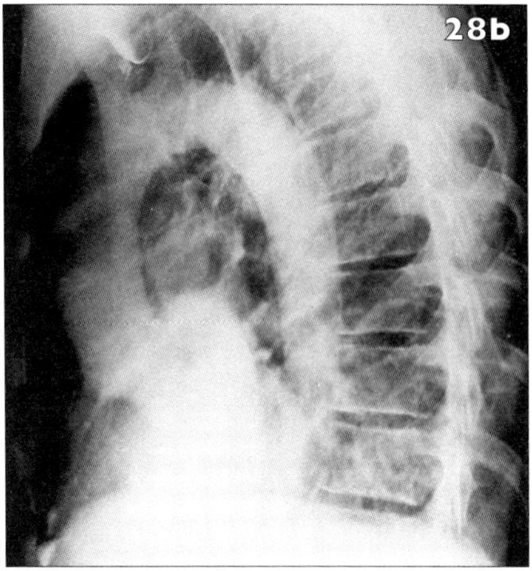

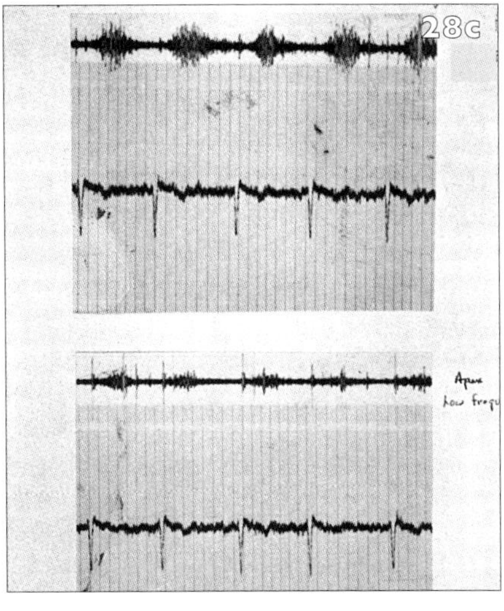

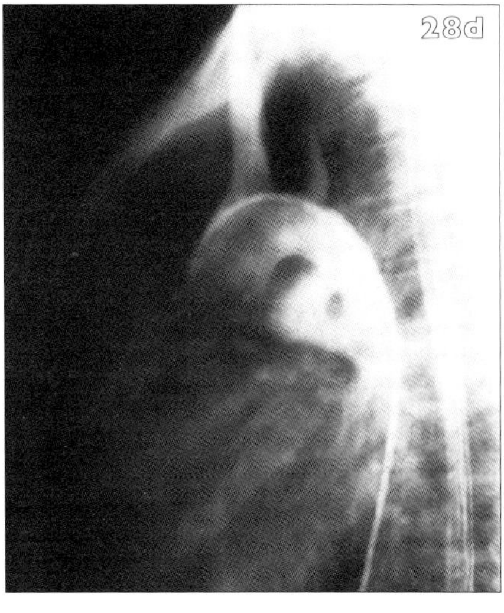

28 A 25-year-old man was found by his family doctor to have a murmur. The family doctor referred him to a hospital cardiologist. A series of investigations produced the images in **28a–28d**.

i. What was the murmur and what is the underlying diagnosis?

ii. What are the treatment options?

29 What are the indications for an automatic implantable cardioverter defibrillator?

28 **i.** The murmur shown in the phonocardiogram (**28c**) is a continuous one, being maximal at the aortic component of the second heart sound and minimal during the first heart sound. It is the 'machinery' murmur of a patent ductus arteriosus. The reason for the continuity of the murmur is that there is a flow of blood through the patent arterial duct in both diastole and systole. (This is no longer the case once pulmonary vascular disease has developed; in these circumstances the murmur is shorter and predominantly diastolic, and P2 is accentuated. The increased trans-mitral flow due to left-to-right shunting may be heard as a mid-diastolic mitral murmur. With shunt reversal, the systolic murmur is yet shorter and an early diastolic pulmonary regurgitant murmur can be heard.) Despite the phonocardiogram, the chest radiographs (**28a, 28b**) are not particularly unusual. The angiogram (**28d**) confirms patency of the arterial duct as contrast flows from the aorta to the pulmonary artery.
ii. The appropriate treatment is elective closure of the patent ductus, either per catheter or at open operation, unless the duct is very small, in which case the only reason to close it would be to remove the risk of endocarditis.

29 Automatic implantable cardioverter defibrillators weigh approximately 200 g. They are implanted under local anaesthetic and sit beneath the rectus sheath on the anterior abdominal wall. They are connected to the heart via transvenous leads in the right ventricular apex and in the superior vena cava. The right ventricular lead senses the arrhythmia and the lead in the superior vena cava acts as a defibrillator. They are useful in cardioverting ventricular tachycardia and fibrillation.

Implantable cardioverters are implanted in patients with sustained monomorphic ventricular tachycardia not caused by myocardial ischaemia, drugs, or electrolyte abnormalities, particularly if the arrhythmias have been evoked during electrophysiological studies in spite of anti-arrhythmic therapy. The other main indication for implantation of the defibrillator is in patients who have recurrent ventricular tachyarrhythmias, accompanied by syncope or profound hypotension, which are not controlled with anti-arrhythmic therapy. Automatic cardioverter defibrillators should not be implanted in patients whose ventricular arrhythmias are not sustained or who have very frequent arrhythmias. In the latter case there would be rapid battery failure, due to recurrent delivery of electric shocks, with considerable discomfort to the patient.

Several large studies have shown that the risk of sudden death in patients receiving the cardioverter device is 2% in one year and 5% after five years. Studies comparing anti-arrhythmic drug therapy with automatic cardiovertor defibrillators in the management of ventricular tachyarrhythmias have shown the latter to be superior in terms of mortality.

30 A 40-year-old man from Kerala, southern India, was reviewed because of fatigue and atypical chest pain present for 1–2 years. No other remarkable features emerged in the history. Physical examination revealed elevation of the venous pressure according to the pattern shown in the middle trace (VP). The ECG revealed left ventricular hypertrophy (LVH) only, the chest radiograph was reported as normal and the blood film was normal. Suggest a diagnosis.

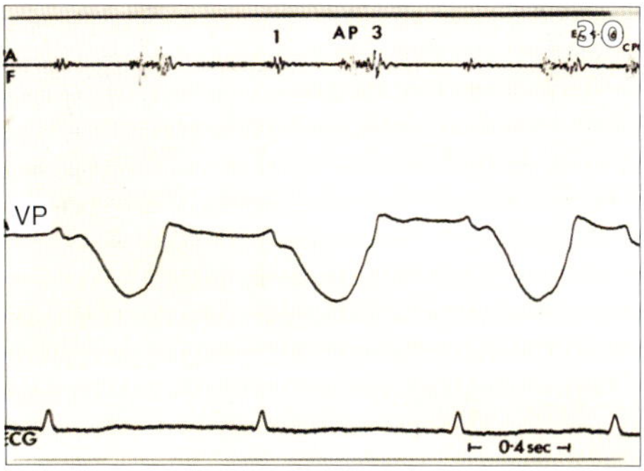

31 A 55-year-old woman with mild breathlessness on exertion suddenly developed severe pain in her right foot. When she presented to hospital, the right leg was cold and pulseless and the great toe was as shown (**31a**). The chest radiograph (**31b**) was performed prior to surgery. In the event, a local anaesthetic was administered and a procedure performed.
i. What is the underlying cardiac disease?
ii. What complication has occurred?
iii. Describe the acute and longer term management.

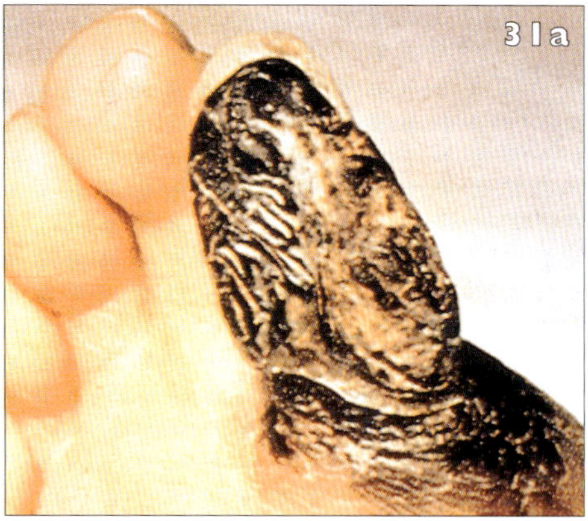

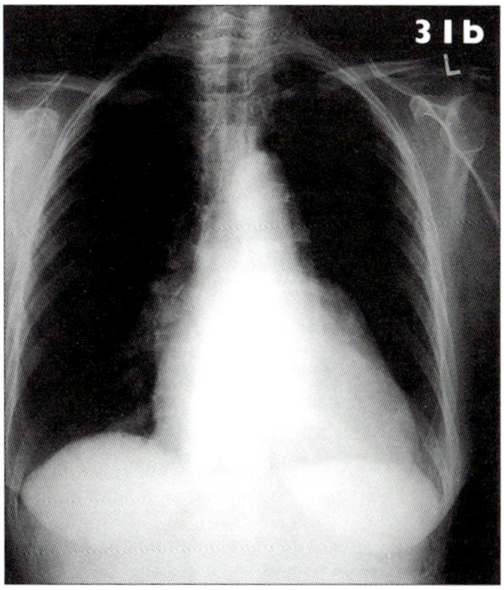

30 Shown is a venous wave form with a raised venous pressure overall, prominent v wave and a rapid y descent. It is typical of restrictive cardiomyopathy. There are several important clues in the question which lead to the diagnosis of tropical endomyocardial fibrosis (EMF). The patient originates from South India. There are no examination findings to suggest constriction (such as a paradoxical pulse). Pericardial effusion is common in EMF, but the heart size remains normal. Both ventricles are involved in the fibrotic process in about half the cases of EMF, with thickening of the right ventricular inflow tract, apex, and papillary muscles, as well as of the tricuspid support structures. On the left, the inflow tract and posterior mitral leaflet are affected. Mural thrombosis with organisation is common in both ventricles; the right apex in particular is obliterated when viewed echocardiographically. Right atrial thrombus is commonly detected. Treatment options other than drug therapy for established heart failure are limited and risky. However, surgical resection of fibrotic endocardium, with mitral valve replacement where appropriate, may be beneficial. The differential diagnosis would include Löffler's syndrome, but the absence of eosinophilia argues against this.

31 **i.** The underlying cardiac disorder is mixed mitral valve disease. The chest radiograph (**31b**) shows the enlarged left atrium and prominent right heart border typical of mitral valve disease.
ii. **31a** shows infarction of the right great toe due to an embolus which has travelled through the left femoral and popliteal arteries before lodging in the relevant digital artery of the foot. (The digital arteries are end arteries.)
iii. The acute management is described in the question. An embolectomy was performed using a Fogarty catheter under local anaesthetic and a clot removed from the right popliteal artery. Subsequent to this, initial anticoagulation with heparin and then oral anticoagulation with warfarin should be instituted, and digoxin administered for control of the ventricular response to the atrial fibrillation. The severity of the mitral valve disease should be assessed by ECG, chest radiograph and echocardiography.

32 A chronically breathless patient was assessed in the outpatient clinic and the ECG (**32a**) and chest radiograph (**32b**) obtained.

i. What is shown and what is the underlying disorder?

ii. What physical signs are specific to this disorder?

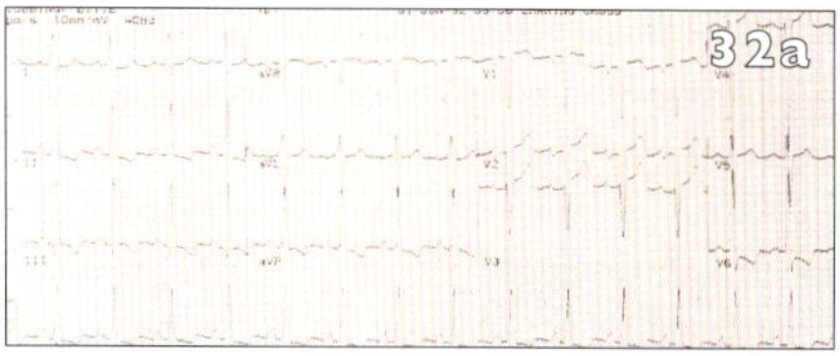

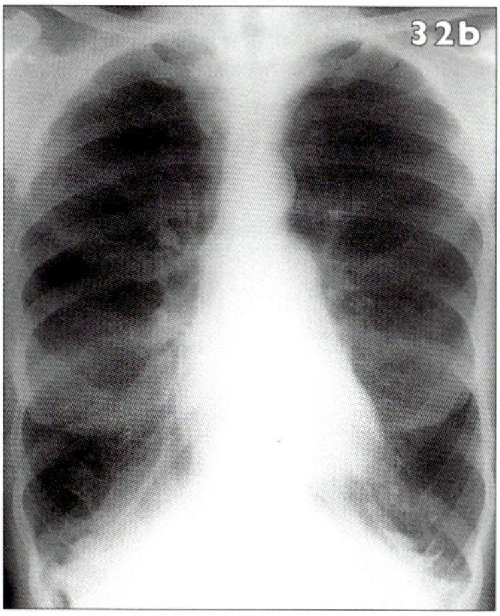

33 What operation has been performed?

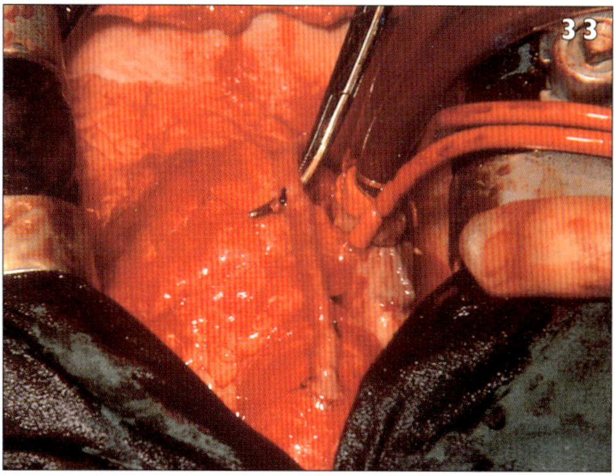

32 **i. 32b** shows hyperinflation of the lungs (attenuation of the peripheral lung fields and flattening of the hemidiaphragms) and an enlarged right heart. The ECG shows right axis deviation, tall P waves ('P pulmonale' – especially in II, III, aVF, and V2), and prominent R waves in V1 and V2, but overall the QRS complexes are small. Investigations into the relationships between these electrocardiographic features and the severity of cardiological or pulmonary functional derangements in this condition have shown right axis deviation to be quite a sensitive index of pulmonary hypertension, but links with the other electrocardiographic signs are tenuous. The findings are typical of chronic obstructive airways disease.

ii. The physical signs include those of hyperinflation of the chest, with tachypnoea and use of the accessory muscles of breathing. Central cyanosis may be detectable if (traditionally) 5 g/dl of reduced haemoglobin is present, a concentration which corresponds to an arterial oxygen saturation of <70% and arterial oxygen tension of about 50 mmHg. Wheezing indicates the presence of bronchoconstriction. Basal crepitations can often be heard, but are *not* necessarily indicative of left ventricular failure. (The Valsalva manoeuvre can help in the clinical distinction of chronic obstructive airways from left ventricular failure – see **164**.) In severe cor pulmonale, signs of right heart failure with tricuspid regurgitation may be elicited.

33 A saphenous vein bypass graft is shown. Coronary artery surgery is recommended for prognostic purposes in patients with either severe three-vessel coronary artery disease or left main stem involvement. Saphenous veins are applied to the ascending aorta and inserted into coronary arteries distal to the diseased segments. The internal mammary artery is now used more frequently and produces a better long-term result. The left internal mammary artery is usually grafted to the native left anterior descending artery and the right internal mammary artery is sometimes used to graft the right coronary artery. The gastroepiploic arteries are now utilised for coronary artery bypass grafting, but the long-term results from these remain to be seen. Saphenous vein grafts have a peri-operative occlusion rate of 10%. Angina recurs in 50% of patients within 5 years. Saphenous vein grafts have a life of approximately 10 years, whereas internal mammary grafts remain patent for much longer. The speed at which the grafts occlude depends a great deal upon whether the patient has poor control over risk factors such as smoking, raised serum cholesterol, and poorly controlled diabetes mellitus.

34 A 40-year-old man complained of angina – his resting ECG is shown in **34a**. A rather inexperienced junior doctor saw him in the outpatient clinic and, having heard a systolic murmur, ordered an echocardiogram (**34b**). Because of the presenting complaint, the doctor also arranged an exercise treadmill test. (AO, Aorta; LV, left ventricle; LA, left atrium; RVOT, right ventricular outflow tract; LVPW, left ventricular posterior wall; IVS, interventricular septum.)

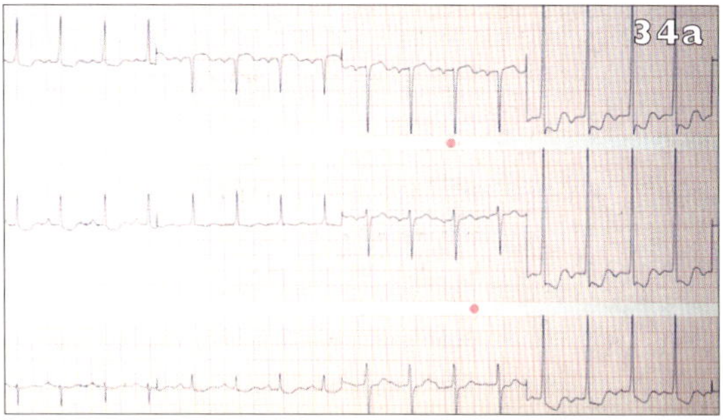
34a

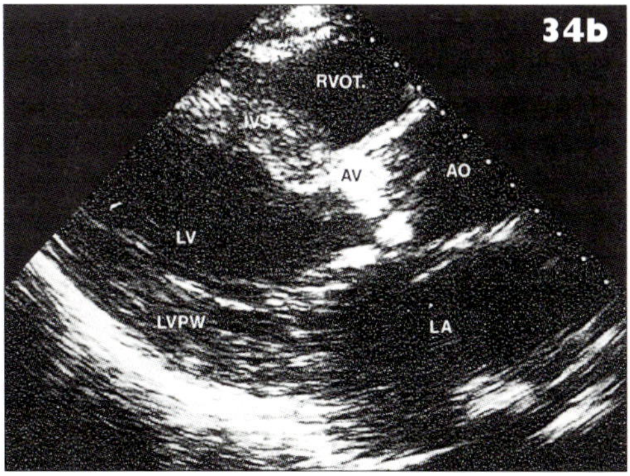
34b

i. What does the echocardiogram show?
ii. What does the ECG show?
iii. What is the diagnosis?
iv. Was the exercise test a good idea?

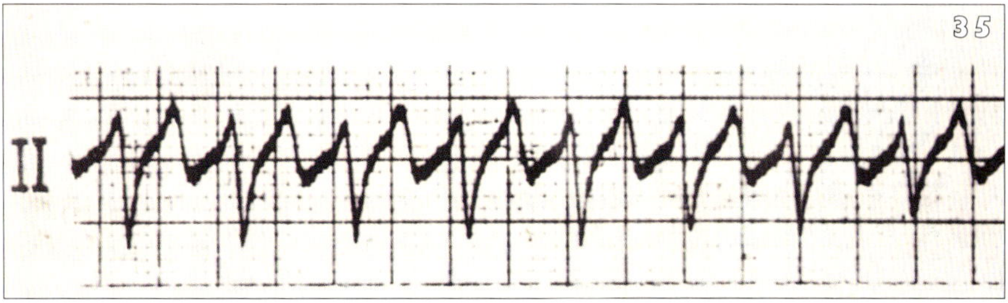
35

35 A 55-year-old employed in a bar found that her work was impaired because of sudden episodes of breathlessness. She consulted her family doctor who recorded this ECG.
i. What is the most likely explanation of the symptom?
ii. How would you treat an acute severe episode?
iii. What further investigations are indicated?

34 i. The echocardiogram (**34b**) shows considerable enhancement of the echoes from the aortic valve, demonstrating thickening and calcification of the valve. There is also reduction in movement of the valve leaflets. The left ventricular wall thickness is greater than normal.
ii. The ECG (**34a**) shows left ventricular hypertrophy with lateral ST segment depression at rest ('strain' pattern).
iii. The underlying diagnosis is aortic stenosis. There is no simple relationship between the measured voltages on the ECG and the trans-aortic gradient, neither is there a clear relationship between the latter and the amount of valve calcification. However, the presence of the strain pattern on the ECG is suggestive of severe left ventricular hypertrophy. Continuous-wave Doppler echocardiography is used to calculate the left ventricular–aortic pressure gradient.
iv. In general, exercise testing is contraindicated in symptomatic aortic stenosis, because of the risks of syncope and arrhythmia. The syncope is at least partially due to inadequate ventricular filling during tachycardia, as well as to left ventricular ischaemia. In addition, baroreceptor activation and peripheral vasodilatation may cause systemic hypotension. Arrhythmias are probably due to ischaemia of the hypertrophied myocardium.

35 i. The ECG shows atrial flutter (note the 'sawtooth' pattern of F waves). Atrial flutter is a re-entrant atrial arrhythmia with an atrial rate of about 300 b.p.m. Typically, a 2:1 atrioventricular block is present, giving a ventricular rate of about 150 b.p.m., as shown. This paroxysmal arrhythmia is responsible for the attacks of breathlessness. The woman is employed in a bar and both increased alcohol consumption and coronary artery disease have an above-average prevalence among this group of workers. Other causes of flutter must be excluded – paroxysmal atrial flutter may occur in the absence of organic heart disease (see **iii**).
ii. In an acute episode of atrial flutter, a low energy DC shock is highly effective. In addition, vagal manoeuvres or adenosine bolus can sometimes reduce the ventricular rate by transiently increasing the degree of atrioventricular block. Several drugs may provide short-term rate control (including digoxin, quinidine, verapamil, beta-blockade, propafenone, flecainide, or amiodarone), either by slowing the flutter rate or increasing the degree of atrioventricular block. However, this arrhythmia tends to be resistant to pharmacological reversion, despite nearly always responding to electrical cardioversion.
iii. Thyroid disease should be excluded. Myocardial ischaemia should be considered, but atrial flutter or fibrillation are not usually caused by it. Echocardiography is of value for the assessment of any underlying structural (including valvar) heart disease.

36 A 70-year-old man was admitted with severe central chest pain, and although his condition was stable for the first 4 days, it declined and he was taken for emergency surgery.
i. What can you see?
ii. How common is this?

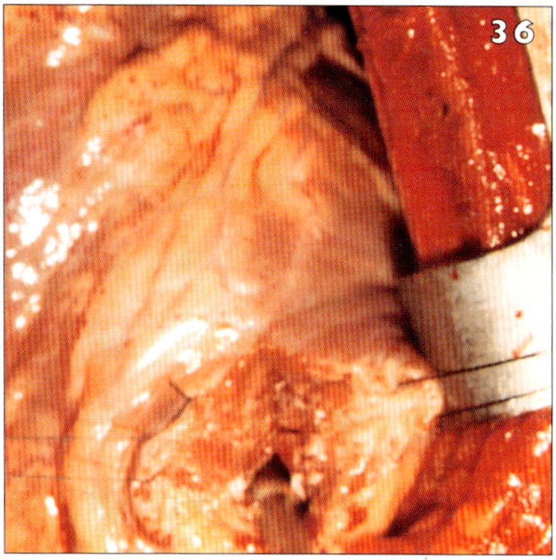
36

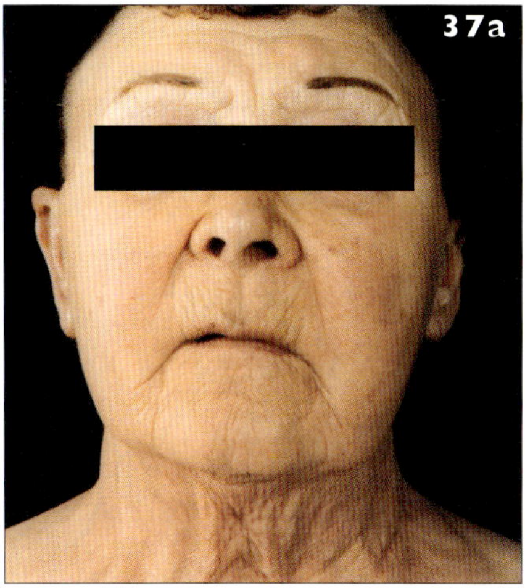
37a

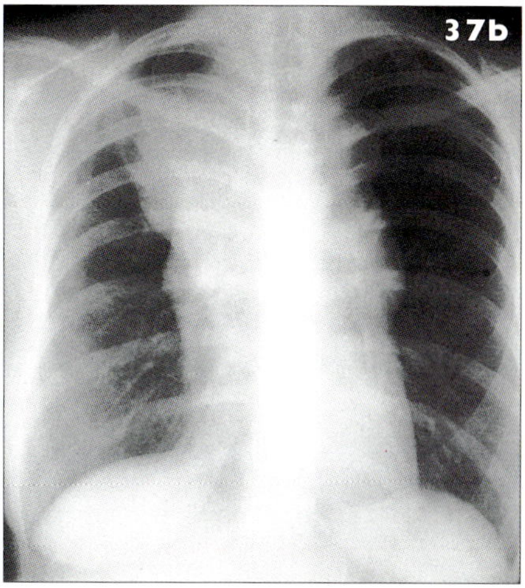
37b

37 This woman recently felt worsening congestion of the head and suffered from headaches, particularly early in the morning. Before this her main complaint was of breathlessness.
i. What is the recent development?
ii. What is the underlying lesion?

36 **i.** The left ventricle of the heart with a fresh infarct is shown; there is a bulge in the infarcted area and at the apex of the bulge the tissues are abnormally thin. There is incipient rupture of the left ventricle in a patient who had an anterior infarct 5 days previously.
ii. Overall, approximately 10% of fatalities after acute myocardial infarction are cases of left ventricular free wall rupture. The majority of these occur within the first 2–3 days after infarction and death is virtually always the outcome, via cardiac tamponade. The rupture develops through a tear at the margin of viable and necrotic myocardium, promoted by the pressure generated during systole and the shear stresses generated by the contraction of viable myocardium in continuity with akinetic tissue. The clinical scenario here is a patient recovering from a myocardial infarction, with infarct expansion and thinning and aneurysm formation. In a few cases, the pathway through the myocardium is indirect, following tissue planes, so that the rupture takes the form of a more gradual leak and slower build up of tamponade than occurs in the rapidly fatal cases. It is in cases like these that there may be an opportunity for a life-saving cardiac surgical intervention. A reduction in the incidence of ventricular rupture after myocardial infarction is one of the benefits of beta-blockers given post myocardial infarction. The incidence of rupture has not been increased by the use of thrombolytic agents. Infarction spreads outwards from endo- to epicardial layers. In limiting infarct size, the epicardial layers tend to be preserved. Both the risk of rupture and the incidence of pericarditis are reduced.

37 Distension of the veins of the neck due to obstruction of the superior vena cava is seen in **37a** – a selective enlargement is shown in **37c** There are several potential causes of this, the most common of which is bronchial carcinoma with local spread. Irradiation of the chest and constrictive pericarditis are also recognised causes. In this case, the chest radiograph (**37b**) shows an aneurysm of the ascending aorta. Thus, the likely sequence of events here is that the gradually enlarging aortic aneurysm eventually produced compression in the superior vena cava. The aneurysm was associated with dilatation of the aortic valve ring, the latter producing valvar regurgitation, left ventricular dilatation, left ventricular failure and breathlessness.

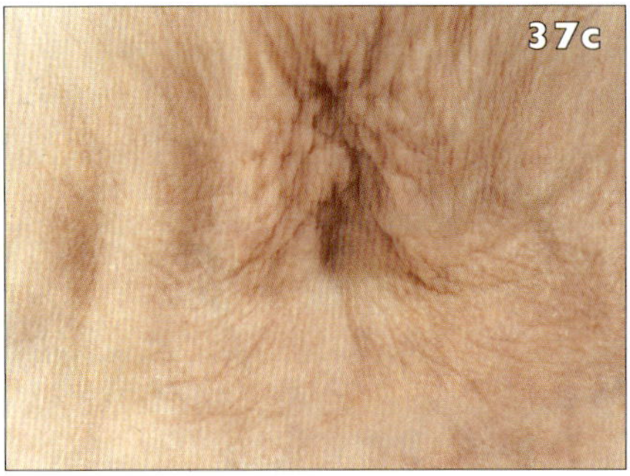
37c

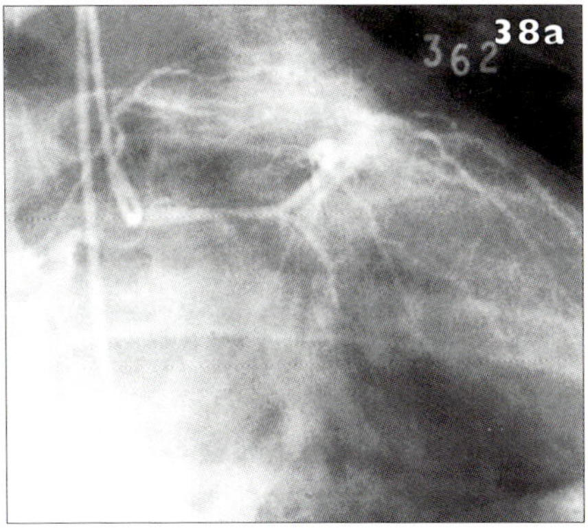
38a

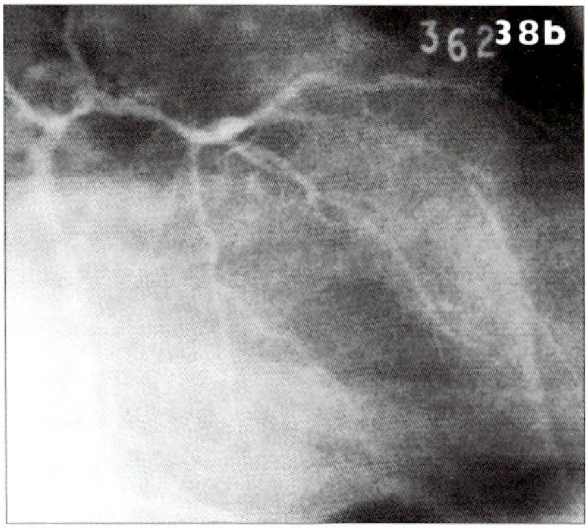
38b

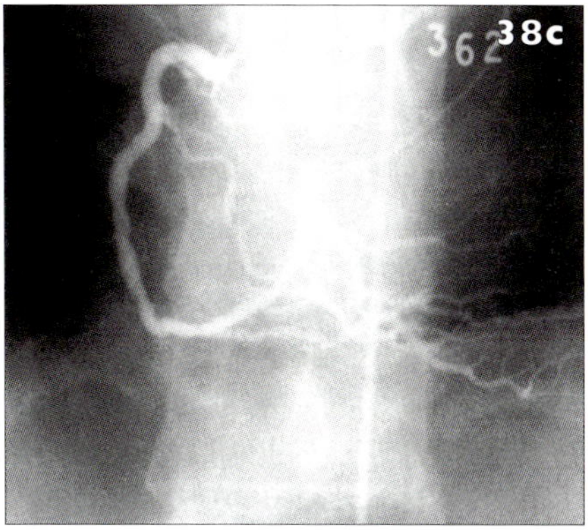
38c

38 Investigations of a 40-year-old man with atypical chest pain produced 38a–38c.

i. What does the arteriogram show?

ii. Does this condition carry any increased cardiovascular risk?

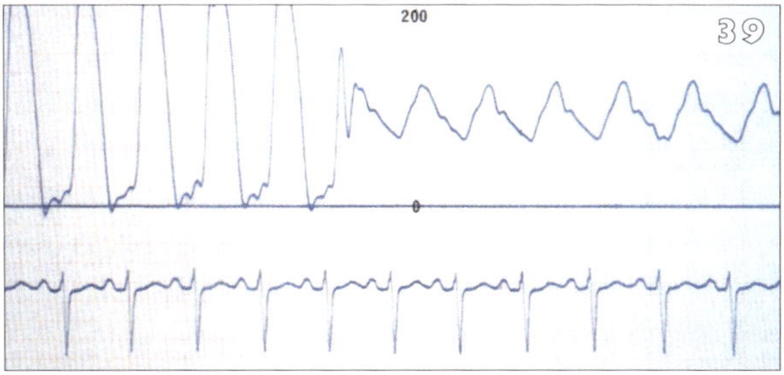

39

39 A 40-year-old man presented with chest pain on exertion.

i. Comment on the pressure trace.

ii. What is the most probable underlying aetiology for the abnormality on the pressure trace?

iii. What is the management?

iv. What may you see during angiography of the left coronary artery?

38 i. This arteriogram shows the left coronary artery (LCA) originating from the right sinus of Valsalva. As far as can be seen from this view, the artery itself is normal.
ii. A number of congenital abnormalities of the coronary arteries are recognised, including anomalous origin of a coronary artery (usually the left) from the pulmonary artery, origin of the left coronary artery (or just its circumflex branch) from the right sinus of Valsalva, origin of the right coronary artery from the left sinus of Valsalva, or hypoplastic coronary arteries and coronary artery–intracardiac shunts (coronary–cameral fistulae). Some of these abnormalities are associated with an increased risk of sudden cardiac death, even in the absence of atheromatous coronary artery disease (CAD). Of the abnormalities listed, the most common is origin of the circumflex from the right coronary sinus, whereas anomalous origin of a coronary artery from the pulmonary artery is the most fatal, often being associated with massive anterior infarction in infancy. In the case shown, with the left coronary artery originating from the right sinus of Valsalva, compression of the anomalous artery between the aortic and pulmonary artery roots, especially when the latter are dilated during exercise, is said to be of pathophysiological significance.

39 i. This is a withdrawal trace from the left ventricle to the aorta. The left ventricular pressure is 200/0 mmHg and the pressure in the aorta is 120/60 mmHg. The peak-to peak gradient across the aortic valve is 80 mmHg. This is an example of moderate-to-severe aortic stenosis.
ii. The most probable cause of aortic stenosis in a relatively young patient is an underlying congenital abnormality of the aortic valve. The commonest such abnormality is a bicuspid aortic valve, present in approximately 1% of the population. The bicuspid valve is exposed to higher turbulent jets in systole than is a three-cusped aortic valve. This leads to calcification of the valve over a period of time, resulting in aortic stenosis. The valve is also prone to infection, so antibiotic prophylaxis is advised during dental work and internal instrumentation (see **180**).
iii. Surgery is recommended as soon as patients develop symptoms.
iv. The left main stem is often short and the circumflex artery is dominant.

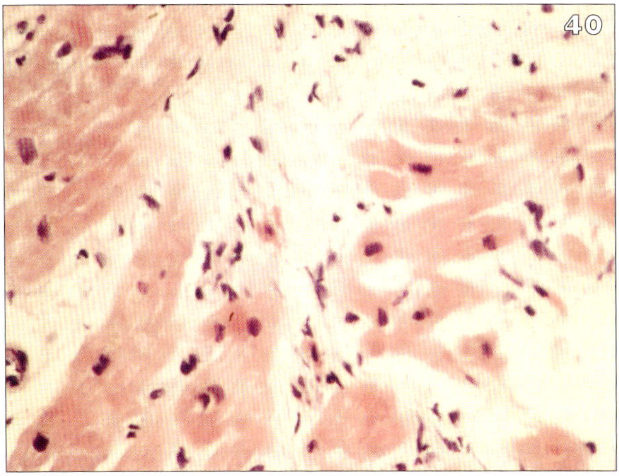

40 A previously fit 21-year-old woman presented with acute heart failure after a few days of a 'flu-like' illness. After stabilisation of her condition, a number of investigations were performed, one of which is shown here.
i. What does the illustration show?
ii. What is the diagnosis and can you be specific?

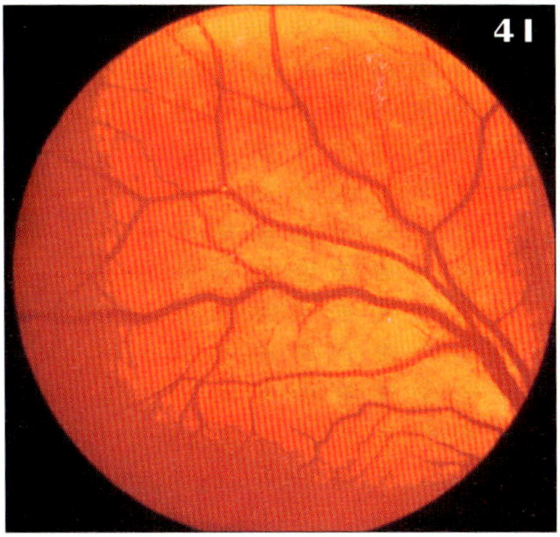

41 A 55-year-old man underwent coronary artery bypass graft surgery, without any apparent complication. However, his wife commented during the first few days after surgery that he was 'just not the same man as he used to be.' Suggest an explanation.

40 i. Shown is infiltration of the myocardium with mononuclear and inflammatory cells and myocytolysis.
ii. The clinical diagnosis is acute (viral) myocarditis. In practice, this is suggested by the preceding viral illness and the presentation with acute heart failure. Typically, there is a wide range of electrocardiographic abnormalities, ranging from varying degrees of heart block (atrioventricular and bundle branch block), atrial and ventricular premature beats, atrial fibrillation, to ventricular tachycardia. Pathological Q waves, ST segment elevation, and T-wave inversion may mimic acute infarction. Chest radiographs and echocardiograms usually show significant dilatation of the chambers of the heart; in addition, a small pericardial effusion may be found. Rising viral titres may be found on serological testing. As far as the biopsy specimen itself is concerned, the microscopic evidence fits the Dallas Myocarditis Panel definition of myocarditis as 'being characterised by an inflammatory infiltrate and by injury to adjacent myocytes that is not characteristic of acute infarction.'
Immunohistochemical staining enables the cells to be identified as T lymphocytes. Viruses have rarely been cultured from biopsy specimens, such as the one shown, and neither have viral antigens been detected, but serological tests may allow the likely causative organism to be identified retrospectively. Any of a very wide range of bacteria, fungi, spirochetes, protozoa, metazoa and rickettsia may be responsible.

41 Shown is a cholesterol embolus in the retinal circulation. Clinically, the patient did undergo a temporary personality change, which was associated with a measurable neuropsychological deficit. This problem is reported to have a prevalence of anything from 1–15% for severe persistent deficits and 5–35% for minor and temporary disturbances. Although the precise mechanism has not been established beyond doubt, a number of hypotheses have been proposed, none of which are mutually exclusive. These include impaired cerebrovascular perfusion during cardiopulmonary bypass due to platelet aggregates, embolisation of thrombus from the left atrium or ventricle, or atheroma from the ascending aortic endothelium. However, previously undiagnosed cerebrovascular disease may be involved, as may thrombosis *in situ* within the cerebral circulation under the circumstances of cardiopulmonary bypass. The tendency in mechanical ventilation to overventilate subjects, thereby making them hypocapnic with associated cerebral vasoconstriction, has also been implicated, as has a potential contribution of reduced cerebral perfusion due to the cardiopulmonary bypass itself (the perfusion pressure of which is about 50 mmHg). Unfortunately, the introduction of finer filters to prevent small emboli, attention to isocapnic ventilation, pulsatile flow from the bypass machine, or increases in perfusion pressure to the brain do not seem to have had much impact upon the overall results.

42 A 65-year-old man presented with acute chest pain, tachycardia and hypotension. What is the diagnosis?

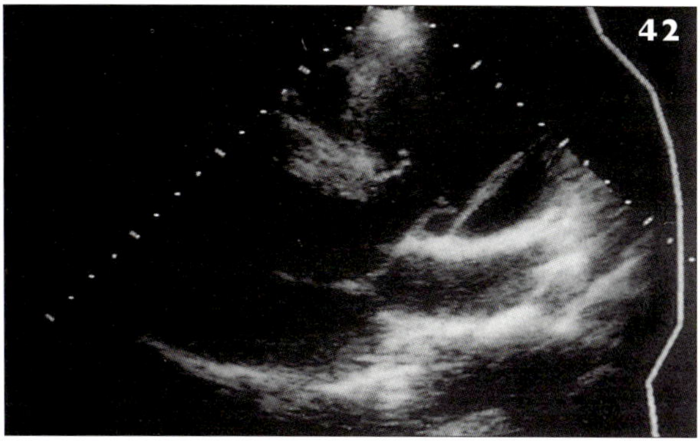

43 This patient presented with breathlessness.
i. What is the underlying diagnosis?
ii. List four possible causes for the breathlessness.

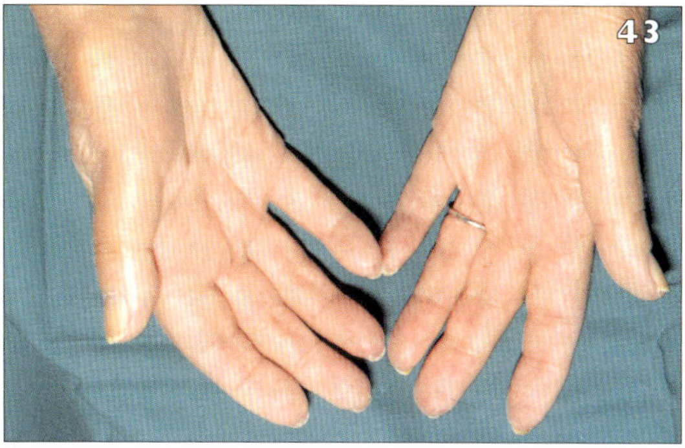

44 What would be the prognosis and management if you observed this tracing in:
i. A 27-year-old asymptomatic professional footballer.
ii. A 54-year-old woman, 5 days after an inferior myocardial infarction.
iii. A 72-year-old man with a year's history of stable angina of effort.

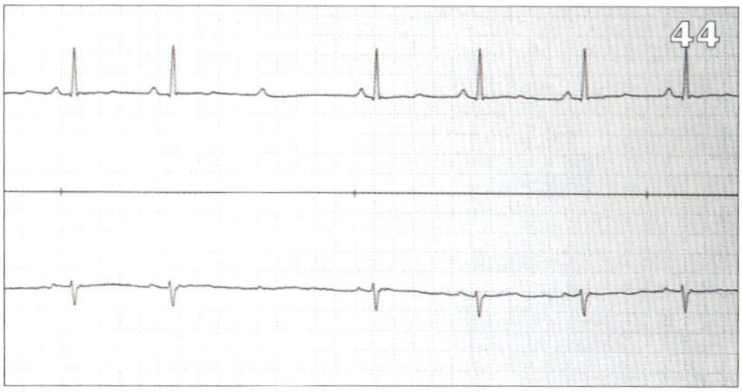

42 This echocardiographic view shows a raised intimal flap quite close to the aortic valve. The valve annulus is symmetrical, but not disrupted, and the aortic dissection is confined to the proximal thoracic aorta; it is therefore a DeBakey type II dissection. This question demonstrates how echocardiography can image the basic lesion in an acute aortic root dissection. Although transthoracic echo may show it, transoesophageal echocardiography is better, with both sensitivity and specificity of the order of 97%. The additional use of colour flow Doppler can permit the localisation of points of communication between the true and false lumina. Echocardiography has revolutionised the diagnosis of proximal aortic dissection and, in most cases, has obviated the need for CT or MR scanning and the previous mainstay of diagnosis, aortography.

43 **i.** The diagnosis is scleroderma. The picture of the hands shows both sclerodactyly and changes consistent with Raynaud's phenomenon.
ii. Possible causes of breathlessness are lung fibrosis, cardiac failure due to cardiomyopathy, pulmonary hypertension, pericardial effusion, heart block, and anaemia.

Systemic sclerosis is a multisystem disorder affecting the skin, kidneys, lungs, gastrointestinal tract and the heart. The disorder has an autoimmune aetiology and is characterised by intimal proliferation within small arteries which lead to necrosis and fibrosis of tissue. Pericarditis is the most common cardiac manifestation and may be complicated by effusions and pericardial constriction. The large epicardial arteries are normal, but angina can occur due to intimal proliferation in the small arterioles. Long-standing ischaemia and necrosis with subsequent fibrosis of myocardial tissue can lead to a myocardial failure. Fibrosis of the conducting tissue can result in various degrees of heart block. Valvar involvement is rare. Hypertension is commonly due to fibrinoid necrosis within the renal glomeruli. Accelerated hypertension is a well-recognised complication of systemic sclerosis.

44 Careful attention to the relationship between the P waves and the QRS complexes in this trace shows that not every P wave is followed by a QRS complex (i.e. conducted to the ventricles). However, there is no gradual increase in the PR interval prior to the non-conducted P wave. This is Mobitz type II atrioventricular (AV) block. The likelihood of progression to complete AV block depends on the clinical context.
i. The 27-year-old professional footballer, free of symptoms, probably has transient type II block due to high vagal tone. He needs no further treatment.
ii. In the case of the 54-year-old woman 5 days after an inferior myocardial infarction, the period of time after the infarct is too long for the AV block to be assumed to be temporary and reversible. She should be monitored for a few days more and then exercised to investigate whether she develops ischaemic changes and, if so, whether this worsens the AV block. Treatment for the ischaemia *per se* may protect against worsening of the AV block. It is very likely that the woman will later need a pacemaker insertion.
iii. Progression to complete heart block is likely in the case of this older patient with established coronary artery disease and pacemaker insertion is necessary.

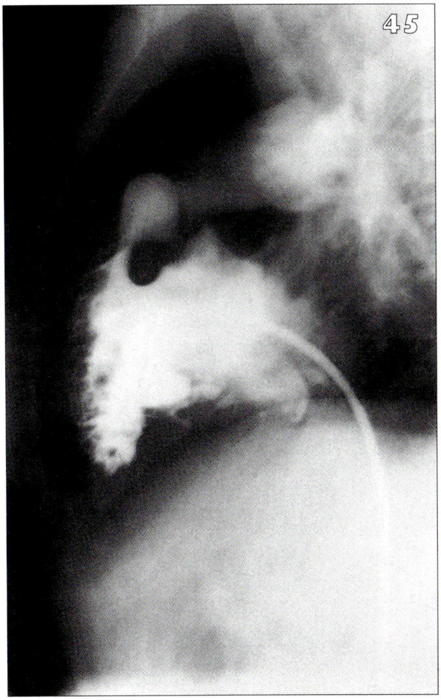

45 A child with the problem shown here underwent a major cardiac surgical procedure.
i. What is the underlying diagnosis?
ii. What definitive procedure could be performed?

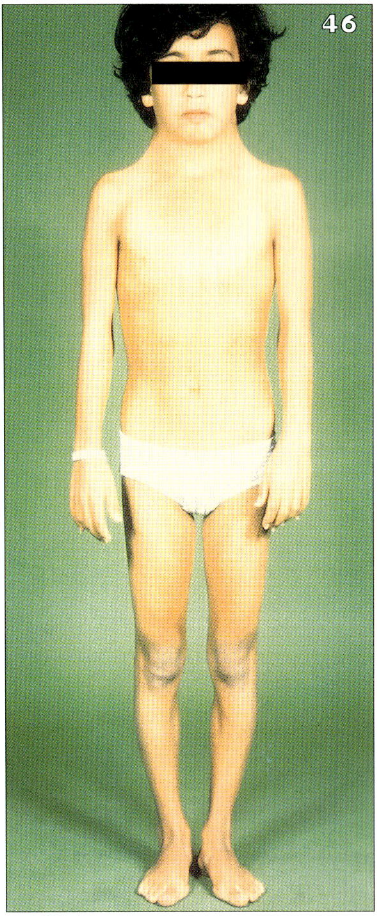

46 This girl has been noted to have a systolic murmur at the second intercostal space to the right of the sternum
i. What is the diagnosis?
ii. What is the murmur due to?

45 i. The angiogram shows the passage of contrast from the right atrium to an enlarged and thickened right ventricle (atrioventricular concordance), and thence into the aorta. There is ventriculo-arterial discordance – the aorta is both anterior and to the right of the pulmonary artery. This characterises complete transposition of the great vessels (TGV). In the example shown there is an associated ASD. Without an associated ASD or VSD, closure of the ductus arteriosus after birth results in a complete separation of the systemic and pulmonary circulations, a situation which is incompatible with life. Prior to ductal closure, cyanosis develops, there is low peripheral vascular resistance, high pulmonary flow, and left ventricular failure supervenes. There is therefore (at least initially) the combination of bounding pulses (high output) and a blue baby (cyanosis). In this particular case, the ASD allowed shunting of a measure of oxygenated blood from the left atrium to the right atrium, thence through the right ventricle and aorta and to the systemic circulation. The time to development of congestive cardiac failure depends inversely on the amount of left-to-right shunting. The combination of TGV and ASD is prognostically one of the best arrangements, children with TGV usually surviving many months unoperated.
ii. Although (a) a prostaglandin infusion can be of value in keeping the ductus temporarily patent in a very cyanosed neonate and (b) a balloon septostomy (Rashkind procedure) can, by enlarging a patent foramen ovale, increase intra-atrial mixing, a definitive procedure is necessary, usually between 6 months and 1 year. Reconstruction at the atrial level (e.g. Senning or Mustard procedures) diverts the pulmonary venous return through the tricuspid valve to the right ventricle and from there to the systemic circulation and, conversely, the systemic venous return from the left atrium via the mitral valve to the left ventricle and from there to the pulmonary artery. The most popular approach currently is the arterial switch operation, performed as early as possible to switch the great arteries to the correct ventricles. If this operation is delayed too long after birth, the left ventricular mass will be too low (due to ejecting into a low pressure system) and will be incapable of sustaining the necessary pressures after the switch. Pulmonary artery banding may be necessary as an interim to evoke left ventricular hypertrophy before the switch operation. Ideally, the infant should undergo total surgical correction in early infancy.

46 i. A phenotypic female with Turner's syndrome is shown. The short stature, webbed neck, and cubitus valgus are characteristic. Turner's syndrome has an incidence of 1/2500 births and is due to the genotypic defect of one X chromosome being absent (45 X0).
ii. Turner's syndrome is associated with coarctation of the aorta in up to 10% of cases. A smaller percentage of patients have congenital aortic valve stenosis. In the girl here, the systolic murmur is due to coarctation of the aorta. Other consistent clinical features would be detectable, such as brachial arterial hypertension and delayed small-volume femoral arterial pulses. Reconstructive surgery for the coarctation is indicated.

47 This is a pathological specimen from a 38-year-old man who complained of polyuria and was being treated for hypertension with a beta-blocker. He was persistently hypokalaemic.
i. What is shown?
ii. How do you account for the polyuria?

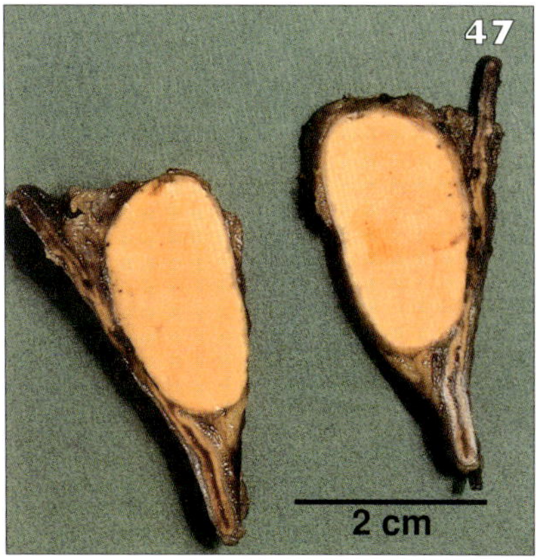

48 A 48-year-old man was admitted to the CCU and an uncomplicated anterior myocardial infarction was diagnosed. His chest pain, however, was troublesome and difficult to manage – in fact, he was not really rid of the pain until 3 days after admission. Explain the pattern of cardiac enzymes shown here.

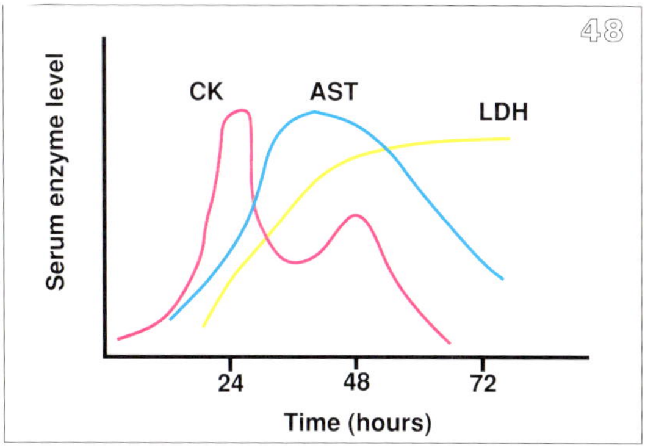

49 A 39-year-old man was admitted with a fever, tachycardia, and breathlessness. He died within 3 hours of admission.
i. What does the heart show post-mortem?
ii. What is the likely responsible organism?

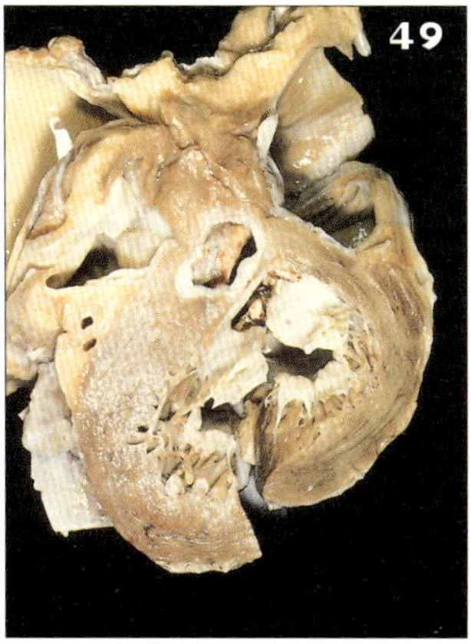

47 i. A macroscopic section of an adrenal gland is shown. There is a firm, yellow, well-defined lesion within the adrenal gland, typical of an adrenal adenoma. The history of hypertension and hypokalaemia fits with either an aldosterone- or a corticosteroid-producing tumour.
ii. The cause of polyuria is either hypokalaemia-induced nephrogenic diabetes insipidus or an osmotic diuresis induced by hyperglycaemia. Patients with primary hyperaldosteronism usually have a mild hypernatraemia, but hyperglycaemia is unusual. Patients with a corticosteroid-secreting adenoma are usually Cushingoid and have hyperglycaemia. The information given here cannot reliably differentiate between the two conditions. An elevated serum aldosterone level in the presence of a suppressed serum renin level would help diagnose primary hyperaldosteronism. An elevated cortisol level which fails to be suppressed by high-dose dexamethasone would diagnose a corticosteroid-producing adenoma. Both conditions are recognised but rare causes of secondary hypertension (see also **178**).

48 The necrosis of cardiomyocytes, which characterises myocardial infarction, permits the release of a number of intracellular enzymes. The principal ones measured are creatine kinase (CK, of which the CK-MB isoenzyme is fairly specific for myocardial necrosis and can be of diagnostic value if the ECG is equivocal), aspartate aminotransferase (AST), and lactic dehydrogenase (LDH, which has five isoenzymes and is sometimes measured as hydroxybutyric dehydrogenase activity, HBD). It is the time course of changes in the levels of these enzymes which, in the context of chest pain and electrocardiographic changes, allows a clinical definition of myocardial infarction. An increase in CK can be detected within about 4 hours of infarction; it peaks between 6–12 hours in the case of early reperfusion after thrombolytic therapy and between 12–24 hours if there is no early reperfusion. AST peaks at about 48 hours and LDH around 72 hours. In the example shown, a second CK peak can be seen about 48 hours after admission, suggesting early reinfarction or that the original episode was of a 'stuttering' nature. Such a patient should, if possible, have been taken to the catheter laboratory and angioplasty of the culprit lesion performed. Recently, cardiac troponin T levels have shown promise for even earlier (earlier than CK-MB) detection of myocardial necrosis.

49 i. The heart shows gross ulceration of the endocardial surface, including of the valves.
ii. The clinical history and gross post-mortem appearances are characteristic of acute pyogenic endocarditis. The most likely cause is *Staphylococcus aureus*. In acute endocarditis, the patient is extremely ill with a fulminant septicaemia and rapid destruction of heart tissues with abscess formation as shown (but often few or only small vegetations) and systemic effects of sepsis, including shock and disseminated coagulopathy (see also **63**).

50 A 56-year-old man was referred to a cardiologist because his blood pressure was 155/95 mmHg and he had also felt his 'heart jumping'. On further questioning, he said he had difficulty sleeping. On examination, his heart rate was 110 b.p.m., regular, and a click and late systolic murmur were heard. Explain the findings and give the diagnosis.

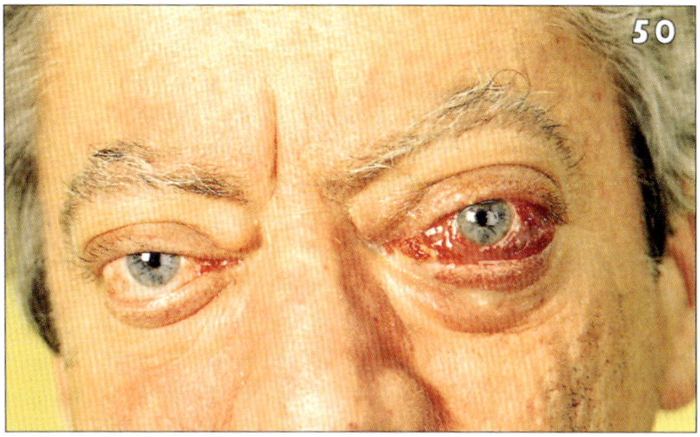

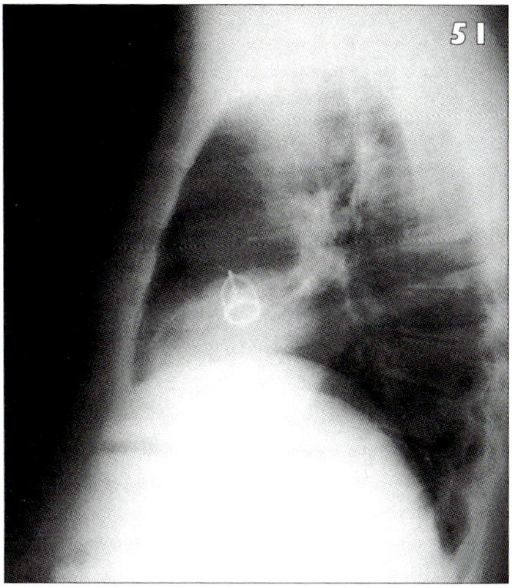

51 i. What does this chest radiograph show?
ii. What are the advantages and disadvantages of this artificial implant?

52 A 63-year-old woman was admitted with pains in all four limbs and with difficulty in lifting heavy objects. She had been seen in clinic six weeks previously and noted to have a serum cholesterol of 8.3 mmol/l (321 mg/dl). The attending doctor commenced her on a statin drug to help reduce the cholesterol level because he was worried about its effects on the coronary arteries, particularly because she was a smoker and also suffered with hypertension. She was a teetotaller. On examination she had tender muscles, her blood pressure was 150/90 mmHg, and serum electrolytes were: sodium, 131 mmol/l; potassium, 6.0 mmol/l; urea, 15 mmol/l (BUN, 42 mg/dl); creatinine 600 μmol/l (6.8 mg/dl).
i. What is the diagnosis?
ii. How can the diagnosis be confirmed?
iii. What is the probable causal agent in this case?

50 The man has obvious exophthalmos; thus the underlying disorder is Grave's disease, i.e. hyperthyroidism due to a circulating auto-antibody to the thyroxine receptor. He had a sinus tachycardia on examination, but had experienced paroxysms of atrial fibrillation, hence the 'heart jumping'. In addition to this, the click and late systolic murmur were due to mitral valve prolapse, a disorder with a reported incidence of up to 30% in patients with hyperthyroidism. More generally, a wide range of cardiovascular symptoms and signs can be found in the hyperthyroid patient, including palpitations, breathlessness, tachycardia, and systolic or even diastolic hypertension. The circulation is typically hyperdynamic with a loud first heart sound and, at times, a third sound. Haemodynamically, cardiac output is increased, as are ejection fraction and velocity of wall shortening. The systolic ejection period is shortened and the pulse pressure widened; peripheral resistance is reduced. However, most of the changes listed are due to increased myocardial contractility, rather than reduced left ventricular afterload. Sinus tachycardia is characteristic of the hyperthyroid state and the heart rate increase is proportional to the disease severity. Paroxysms of atrial fibrillation are common and persistent atrial fibrillation readily becomes established. Less commonly, atrioventricular conduction defects are found in thyrotoxicosis, as are supraventricular tachycardia and atrial flutter. In severe untreated thyrotoxicosis, cardiac failure can ensue.

51 **i.** The chest radiograph shows a Starr–Edwards valve in the mitral location – both the ball and the cage of the prosthetic valve can clearly be seen.
ii. As with other mechanical valve prostheses, life-long anticoagulation is required in patients with a Starr–Edwards valve prosthesis. In addition, the development of a paravalvar leak can cause appreciable haemolysis. Haemodynamically, there might be a greater degree of residual functional stenosis with the Starr valve than with tilting disc prostheses, especially in patients with a small left ventricular cavity. However, this is offset by a long track record of durability. Levels of anticoagulation used now are lower than formerly, which has reduced the risk of bleeding while not increasing the thromboembolic risk.

52 **i.** The history of muscular pain, evidence of renal impairment with disproportionate elevation of the serum creatinine when compared to the serum urea, point to the diagnosis of rhabdomyolysis.
ii. The diagnosis can be confirmed by finding an elevated serum creatinine phosphokinase and by the estimation of urinary myoglobin.
iii. The most probable cause of rhabdomyolysis in this case is treatment with the statin drug. The statins are extensively used for the treatment of hypercholesterolaemia and are very effective drugs in this situation. Very rarely they can cause a myositis, which can precipitate renal failure from the toxic effects of myoglobin on the renal tubules. This complication is more likely when statins are used in conjunction with fibrates for the management of hypercholesterolaemia. Management involves withdrawal of the drug and a forced diuresis with central venous monitoring. If the patient becomes oliguric or the creatinine continues to rise then dialysis may become necessary.

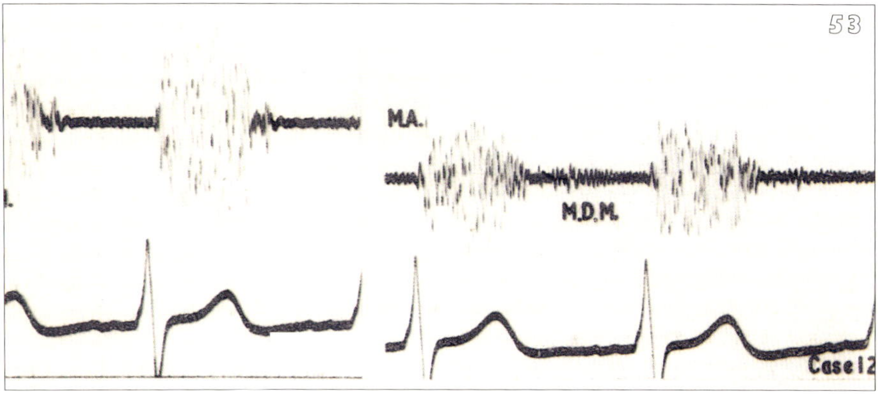

53 **i.** What is this investigation, performed on a young woman, mildly breathless on exertion ?
ii. What does it depict?
iii. Suggest an underlying disorder.

54 This investigation was performed upon a 28-year-old teacher who complained of fluttering episodes in the chest. On further questioning, she also admitted to occasional panic attacks, fainting attacks and chest pain.
i. What does this investigation show and what is the diagnosis?
ii. What are the physical signs specific to this condition?

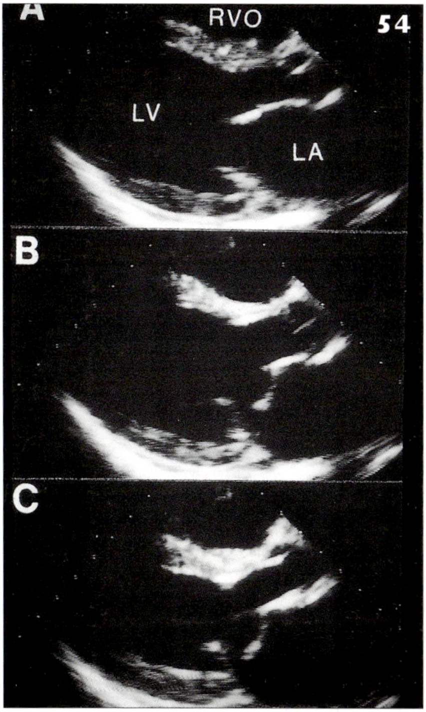

53 **i.** The investigation is a phonocardiogram, recorded at the left sternal edge.
ii. There is a loud medium-pitched pan-systolic murmur.
iii. The underlying disorder is a restrictive ventricular septal defect (VSD). The nature of the added sounds in cases of VSD can convey useful clinical information about the condition. Thus, in a small VSD, the murmur is usually a harsh pan-systolic one, heard maximally around the left side of the sternum, third intercostal space. The murmur may not be pan-systolic if the VSD is in the muscular septum and closes during systole due to the contraction of the heart. Conversely, it may terminate during systole because of shunt reversal due to pulmonary hypertension. The aortic component of the second heart sound is usually buried in the systolic murmur. With large left-to-right shunts, a left ventricular third heart sound may be audible, as well as a mid-diastolic murmur due to the increased trans-mitral flow. In patients with large non-restrictive defects, an ejection systolic murmur is heard due to increased flow through the pulmonary valve, and the pulmonary component of the second heart sound is loud. In patients with severe pulmonary vascular disease flow murmurs are absent. There may be an ejection click, the second sound is 'single' (due to synchronous pulmonary and aortic valve closure) and a pulmonary regurgitant end-diastolic murmur may be heard.

54 **i.** This 2D echo trace (parasternal long-axis view) shows three views of the cardiac cycle from diastole to systole (A to C). The posterior mitral leaflet can be seen to prolapse during late systole, i.e. when the left ventricular chamber size is at its smallest. The patient has mitral valve leaflet prolapse syndrome (see 87); her clinical history includes a number of the clinical features of this condition – palpitations (mainly ventricular ectopic beats during exercise), atypical chest pain, and an increased incidence of panic disorder. The prevalence of this disorder is greatest in younger, female patients.
ii. The physical signs typically comprise a mid-systolic click and a late systolic mitral regurgitant murmur (the latter may not be present). The greater the redundancy of mitral valve tissue, the earlier the click is heard in the cardiac cycle; also characteristic is that the auscultatory features vary with posture. The click (or clicks) and murmur start earlier when the patient stands up and later when the patient lies down or squats, due to changes in left ventricular volume.

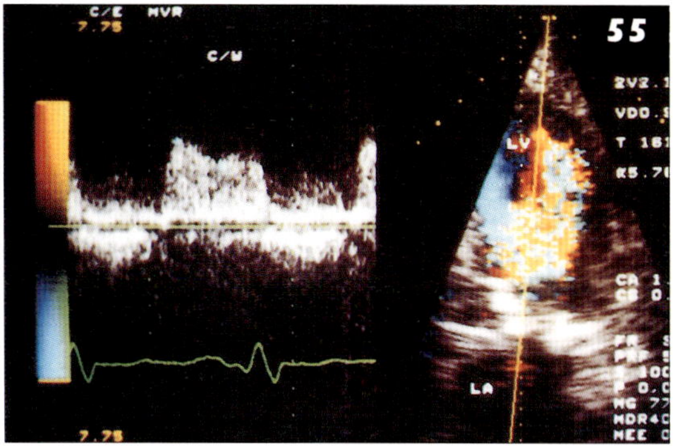

55 This investigation was performed upon a 50-year-old woman who had experienced breathlessness on exertion for a number of years, but this had worsened in recent weeks.
i. What is the investigation?
ii. What is the diagnosis?
iii. Can you derive any quantitative anatomical information from the velocity data?

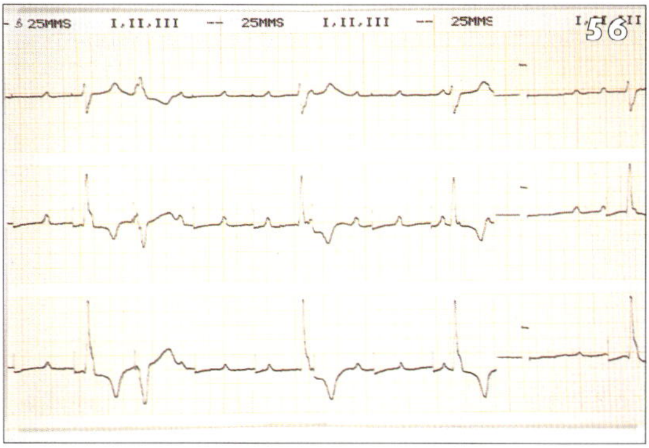

56 The trace was taken during a pacing check, which was performed earlier than planned because this patient (who has a permanent pacemaker *in situ*) developed dizzy spells. What is the cause of her dizzy spells?

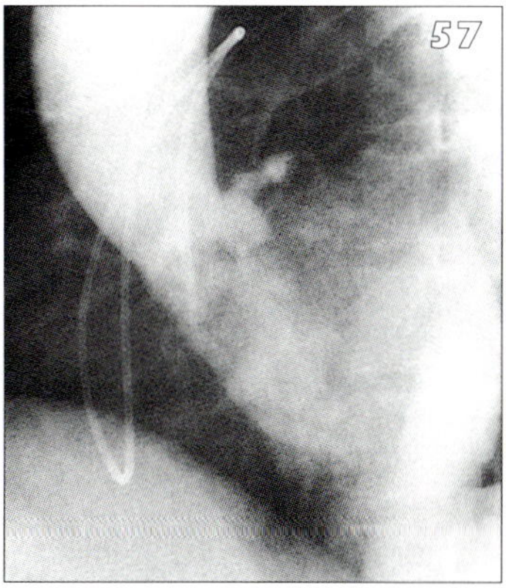

57 A 42-year-old man had complained of lower back pain on and off for 5 years. Since a number of his relatives habitually complained of the same problem he tended to ignore it. In the end, however, he was persuaded to undergo assessment by a hospital physician. The physician referred him to a cardiologist and eventually he underwent the investigation shown.
i. What does the investigation show?
ii. What is the underlying diagnosis?
iii. What are the genetic implications?

55 **i.** This is a continuous-wave Doppler study.
ii. The 2D part of the slide shows that the Doppler sampling of velocity is across the mitral valve. The wave form is characteristic of mitral stenosis. There is no late diastolic velocity increase, since the patient is in atrial fibrillation and the atrial filling phase has been lost.
iii. In atrial fibrillation several (i.e. at least ten) beats must be recorded before it can be assumed that a representative value of the pressure half-time has been obtained. With this proviso, the mitral valve area can be estimated on the basis of the equation:

$$\text{valve area (cm}^2\text{)} = 220/\text{pressure half time (ms)}$$

Accurate numerical values of velocity can be obtained using continuous-wave Doppler (see **102**). Although pulsed wave Doppler is capable of recording the increased flow velocity found across a moderately stenotic mitral valve, there is a problem at higher flow velocities due to aliasing (i.e. a 'wrapping round' of the highest velocities to the lowest end of the velocity scale, due to the limit that sampling of pulses of velocity places upon the maximum frequency shifts detectable).

56 The patient has a ventricular pacemaker. The underlying rhythm is complete atrioventricular dissociation. Pacing spikes are seen to occur at a rate of 75 per minute; however, there is failure to capture and depolarise the ventricular myocardium. If the pacemaker was functioning correctly the pacing spikes would be followed by a wide QRS complex representing ventricular depolarisation and contraction. The dizzy spells are due to a very low heart rate and, consequently, a low cardiac output. The most common cause of failure to capture is lead displacement. An increase in the threshold of the myocardium can also cause this problem, as can too low an output voltage. In this situation the ventricular lead needs to be tested and then either repositioned or replaced.

57 **i.** This is an aortogram which shows opacification of the whole of the left ventricular chamber during diastole. This is aortic regurgitation of grade III severity – the contrast fills the ventricle, but empties each systole. (Grade I regurgitation refers to dye which just flows back into the ventricle; in Grade II severity, regurgitant dye gradually fills the entire left ventricular chamber, and Grade IV regurgitation describes the situation of contrast filling the ventricle in one diastole, but never being cleared in systole.)
ii. The inherited cause of back pain suggests an underlying diagnosis of ankylosing spondylitis. A recognised association of ankylosing spondylitis is aortitis, of which the aortic regurgitation is a complication.
iii. Tissue typing of this patient revealed him to be positive for HLA B27. The strong association of ankylosing spondylitis with HLA B27 means that any relative with the same histocompatibility typing would be about 100 times more likely to develop ankylosing spondylitis than the general population.

58 A 70-year-old woman was investigated for 'dizzy spells'.
i. What can you conclude from the ECG?
ii. How should the woman be treated and what are the complications of such treatment?

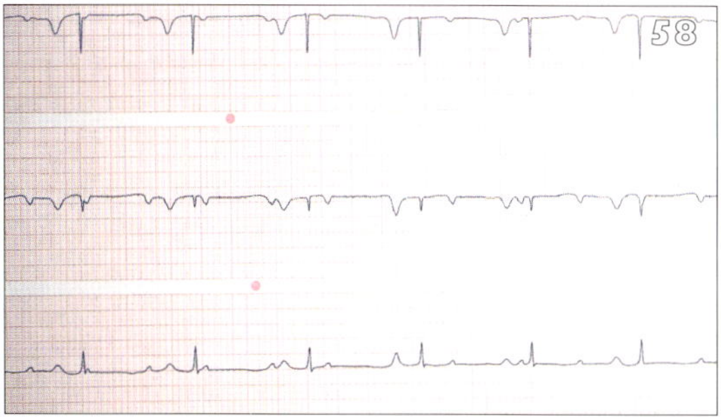

59 This 72-year-old man on treatment for heart failure presented with nausea and intermittent palpitations.
i. Define the rhythms in (A), (B), and (C).
ii. Which two investigations would you request?
iii. What is the cause of his symptoms?

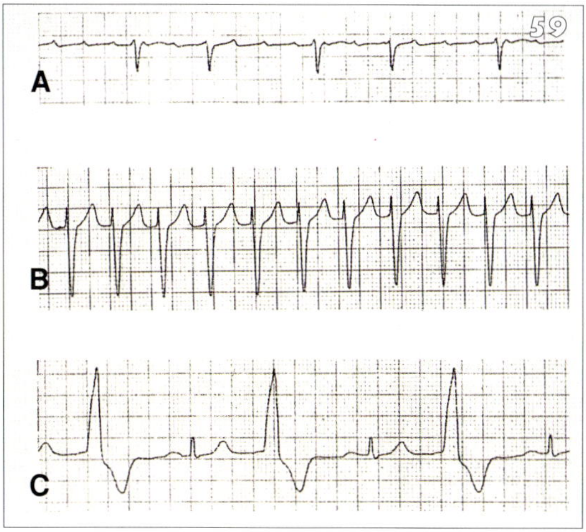

60 In this diagram of the conduction pathways through the atrioventricular node, predict the ECG consequences of conduction down the pathways marked A, B, and C.

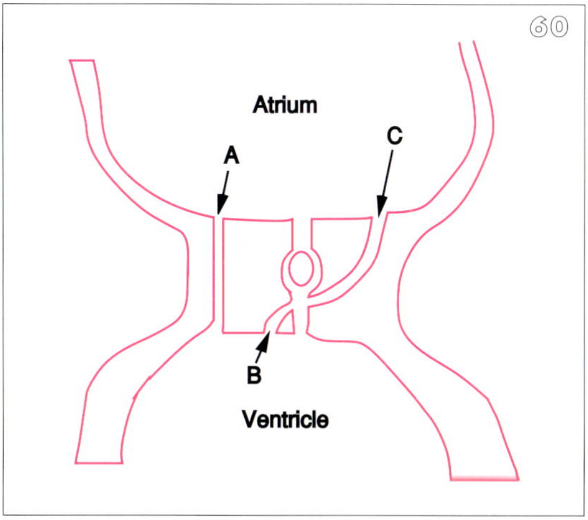

58 **i.** The ECG shows complete dissociation between the P waves and QRS complexes, i.e. they are asynchronous. The prolonged pauses between ventricular contractions caused the dizzy spells. If sufficiently prolonged, so as to result in collapse, these are Stokes–Adams attacks.
ii. The treatment of this condition is insertion of a permanent pacing system. The simplest is a demand ventricular pacing system (VVI mode). The theoretical ideal to produce a more physiological cardiac cycle, responsive to the needs of exercise, would be a dual chamber system (DDDR mode). The complications of pacemaker insertion include infection of the pacemaker pocket, lead displacement or penetration of the ventricle with failure to capture or loss of sensing; both of these can produce dizziness or missed beats. Dizziness and syncope can follow from myoinhibition, in which a 'false' signal from the pectoral muscles inhibits pacemaker activity. Late lead fracture produces a recrudescence of the pre-implantation symptoms. The so-called pacemaker syndrome, which includes dizziness and heavy palpitations, is caused by atrial distension after retrograde conduction to the atrium. It is prevented by dual chamber pacing.

59 The rhythms are (A) complete heart block, (B) atrioventricular nodal tachycardia, and (C) ventricular bigemini.
ii. Serum digoxin and serum potassium levels should be obtained.
iii. The most likely cause of the symptoms is digoxin toxicity. The most common symptoms of digoxin toxicity are nausea, anorexia and vomiting. Xanthopsia is a classic symptom, but is very rare. Cardiac arrhythmias occur, the most common being ventricular ectopics and ventricular bigemini. Other arrhythmias include paroxysmal atrial tachycardia, second or third degree block, ventricular tachycardia, and junctional bradycardia. Digoxin toxicity is often precipitated by hypokalaemia and, because most patients who take digoxin also take diuretics, this is a relatively common scenario. Other factors that predispose to toxicity are hypomagnesaemia, hypercalcaemia, hypoxia and hypothyroidism.

60 **i.** A indicates the Bundle of Kent. In this situation – that of classical Wolff–Parkinson–White syndrome – the accessory bundle is entirely separate from the atrioventricular node. It traverses the atrioventricular fibrous ring completely. Therefore, on the ECG the PR interval is shortened and a ∂ wave is present.
ii. B indicates Mahaim fibres. This accessory pathway arises in the atrioventricular node or His bundle and ends in the ventricular myocardium. The PR interval tends to be normal as only part of the nodal pathway is bypassed. If the fibre terminates on the His bundle, then a ∂ wave may be seen.
iii. C indicates James fibres. These accessory pathways are either intranodal or intrafascicular bypass tracts. On the ECG, a short PR interval with a normal QRS complex is to be expected. In association with paroxysmal tachycardia, this constitutes the Lown–Ganong–Levine syndrome.

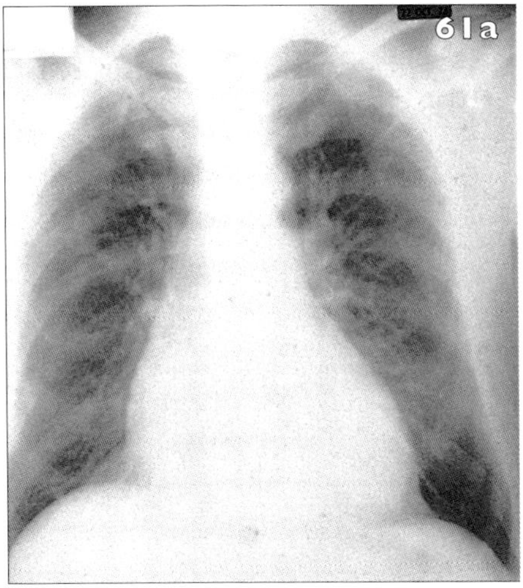

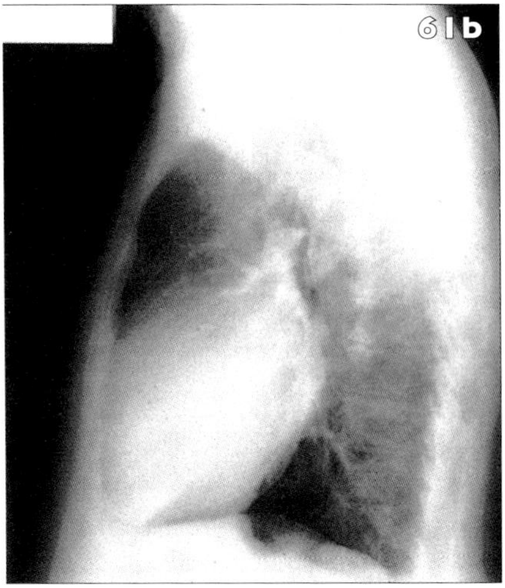

61 A 50-year-old jazz pianist complained of increasing breathlessness on exertion in the absence of chest pain. His coronary arteries were reported as having only minimal disease. Suggest, on the basis of the chest radiographs (**61a**) and (**61b**), a diagnosis, a mechanism for it, and the outlook.

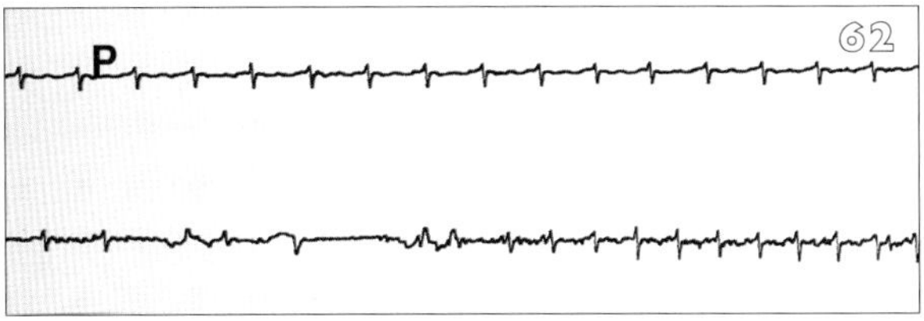

62 A 46-year-old male presented to emergency department feeling breathless and dizzy. An ECG strip showed the rhythm illustrated here. At point P a bolus injection of adenosine was given. (*NB* The second line of the tracing is the continuation of the first.)

i. What was the presenting rhythm?

ii. What has been achieved by the injection?

iii. What is the mechanism of action of adenosine and what are the side effects?

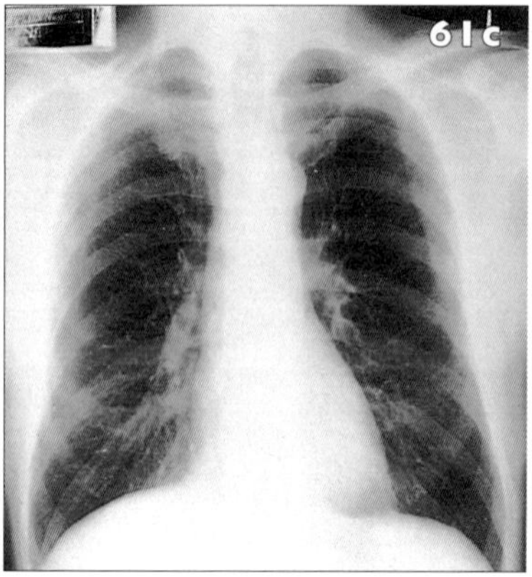

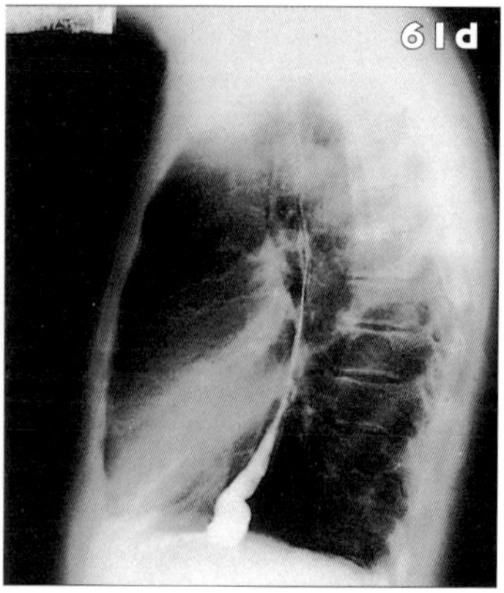

61 This jazz musician steadily drank 10–15 units of alcohol each night during his recitals. He developed alcoholic cardiomyopathy, hence his breathlessness on exertion and dilated left ventricle shown on the upper chest radiograph. The mechanism of alcoholic cardiomyopathy has not been fully elucidated; it may be mediated by a direct toxic action of ethanol on the cardiomyocyte. Alcohol has been shown to inhibit mitochondrial respiration via inhibition of enzymes of the citric acid cycle. It also affects sarcoplasmic uptake of calcium, but the latter effect is not specific, being found in other types of heart failure. Complete abstention from alcohol can be followed by marked improvement [as shown in the chest radiographs (**61c**) and (**61d**)], with a possible 80% likelihood of long-term survival. Further consumption, however, leads to further myocardial deterioration.

62 i. The presenting rhythm was atrioventricular nodal re-entrant tachycardia (AVNRT). There are narrow complexes, all QRS complexes are preceded by P waves, and P waves can also be seen superimposed upon the T wave (as well as coincident with the T waves).
ii. The injection has terminated the run of tachycardia. After 14 beats there are a couple of (probably) aberrantly conducted supraventricular beats followed by a sinus pause, a further couple of aberrantly conducted supraventricular or ventricular ectopics beats, atrial flutter for four beats, and then sinus rhythm.
iii. Adenosine has become the drug of choice in the treatment or unmasking of acute supraventricular tachycardia. It blocks anterograde conduction through the atrioventricular node, but lacks the hypotensive, negative inotropic effect which can make verapamil fatal in ventricular tachycardia. Adenosine also (in contrast to verapamil) does not remove retrograde concealed penetration of the accessory pathway in Wolff–Parkinson–White syndrome, an effect of verapamil which may promote the very rapid and dangerous ventricular response to atrial fibrillation in that condition. Adenosine has an extremely short half life (10–30 s) and is administered by fast intravenous bolus injection of 3, 6, or up to 12 mg.

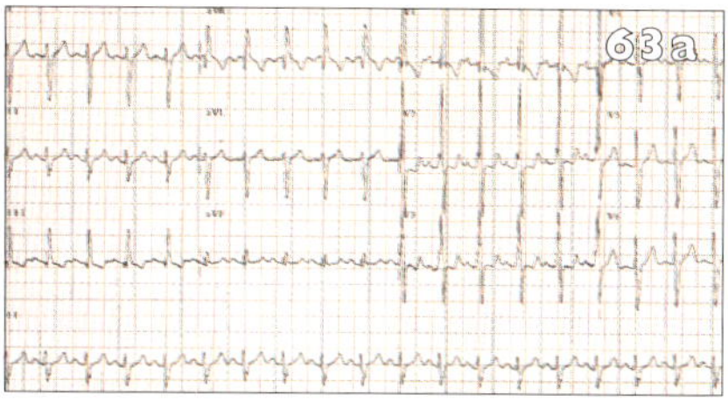

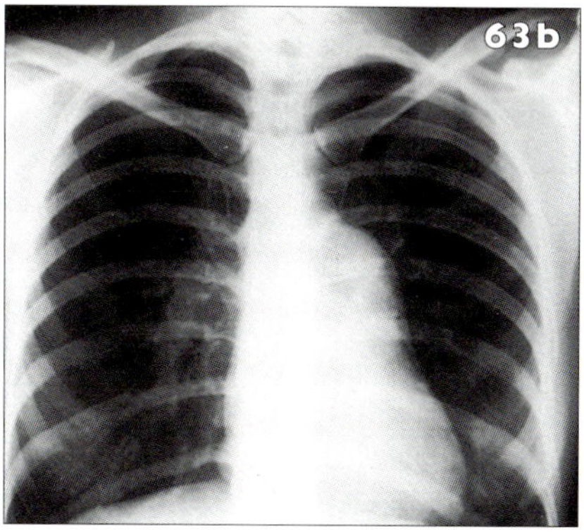

63 A 54-year-old woman was admitted with a 4-day history of a non-productive cough and increasing dyspnoea. She had suffered with recurrent lower respiratory tract infections for several years. She also reported intermittent palpitations during which she experienced no other symptoms. There was no other past medical history of note. She was a smoker. On examination she appeared unwell and was clubbed and peripherally cyanosed. Heart rate was 110 b.p.m., blood pressure 105/70 mmHg, and JVP elevated, but her temperature was not raised. The apex was not displaced, but there was a prominent left parasternal heave. Cardiac auscultation revealed a soft ejection systolic murmur in the pulmonary area, with a loud pulmonary component to the second heart sound. Auscultation of the lung fields was normal.

i. List two abnormalities on the ECG (**63a**).

ii. List three abnormalities on the chest radiograph (**63b**).

iii. What is the probable diagnosis?

iv. Which investigation would you request next?

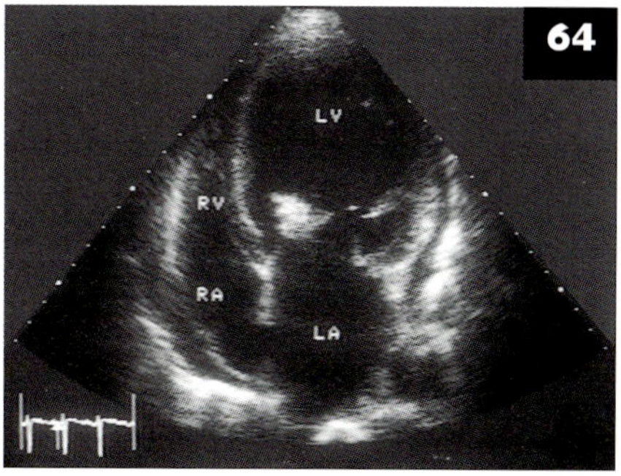

64 This is a transthoracic echocardiogram of a 43-year-old alcoholic who presented with severe pain and loss of power of the left lower limb. For one month he had experienced night sweats, his appetite was reduced, and he had lost several kilograms in weight.

i. What does the echocardiogram demonstrate?

ii. What was the cause of pain in the left leg?

iii. Which two further tests are required?

63 **i.** The ECG reveals rightward axis and partial right bundle branch block. The deep S waves in leads V5 and V6 are suggestive of right ventricular hypertrophy.
ii. The chest radiograph reveals cardiomegaly, enlarged pulmonary arteries, and pulmonary plethora.
iii. The most probable diagnosis is an ostium secundum atrial septal defect (ASD) with secondary pulmonary hypertension.
iv. The next investigation of choice would be a transthoracic echocardiogram to confirm the clinical suspicion and to estimate the size of the defect. In the secundum ASD defect the differential diagnosis is with mild pulmonary stenosis. With the development of pulmonary hypertension the differential diagnosis includes mixed mitral valve disease and cor pulmonale.

64 **i.** A large vegetation is seen on the anterior mitral valve leaflet.
ii. Iliofemoral embolism was the cause of the leg pain.
iii. Six sets of blood cultures and culture of the clot after embolectomy are required.

The diagnosis is endocarditis; although it usually occurs on abnormal valves, endocarditis may affect normal valves. Common pathogens include *Streptococcus viridans*, which is a normal oral commensal. *Staphylococcus aureus* and epidermis infections account for 25% of cases. Fungal endocarditis occurs in the immunosuppressed and in intravenous drug abusers. Other causes include *Coxiella burnetii*, Chlamydia species, Brucella and anaerobic gram-negative bacilli. The patient exhibits signs of infection with fever, chills and night sweats. A murmur is almost always present, with the exception of right-sided endocarditis in which the pressures are often too low to generate murmurs. Signs of immunological activation are present and include splinter haemorrhages, Roth spots, haematuria due to focal segmental glomerulonephritis, and a vasculitic rash. Emboli occur in a third of patients and can affect the central nervous system, limbs and spleen.

Diagnosis is based on clinical suspicion, fever, murmur, positive blood cultures, and echocardiographic evidence of vegetations. Note that small vegetations below 3 mm in size will not be detected by transthoracic echocardiography. Blood cultures are positive if prior antibiotics have not been prescribed. If cultures are negative in the absence of antibiotics, serology should be requested to try and detect any of the other causes of endocarditis, mentioned above.

Treatment involves appropriate antibiotics. The duration of antibiotics is dependent on the organism, sensitivity and response. For the first 2–4 weeks antibiotics are administered intravenously. (See also **194**.)

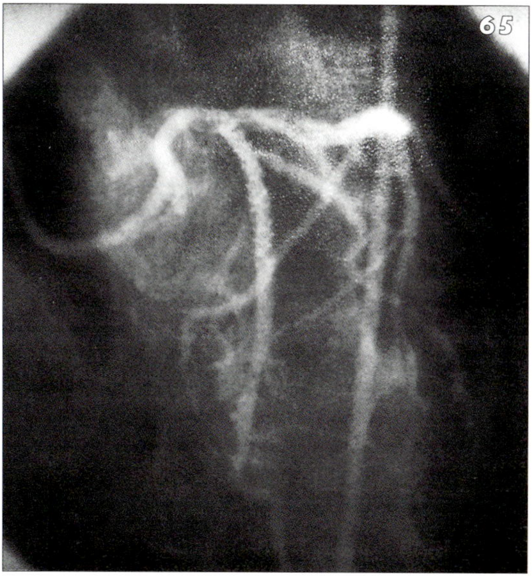

65 This 55-year-old man presented with worsening angina of effort and an exercise stress test revealed ischaemic changes in the anterolateral leads. He underwent coronary arteriography and an angioplasty was performed. After 2 months, however, the pain returned and the whole cycle was repeated. Again, the pain returned after about 2 months.

i. What has happened?
ii. How common is this and how does it occur?
iii. What was done after the two failed angioplasties?

66 An 18-year-old girl complained of increasing breathlessness on exertion. Her cardiac catheterisation data (pressures and saturations) are presented here.

Chamber	*Pressure (mmHg)*	*Chamber*	*O_2 saturation (%)*
Pulmonary capillary wedge (mean)	32	Pulmonary artery	80
Pulmonary artery	91/42	Right ventricular outflow tract	82
Right ventricle	92/20	Mid right ventricle	83
Right atrium	a 14; v 20	Low right atrium	83
Left atrium	a 15; v 22	High right atrium	70
Left ventricle	140/24	Superior vena cava	59
Aorta	138/70	Inferior vena cava	57
		Left ventricle	94

i. What are the diagnoses?
ii. What do you expect her ECG to show?
iii. Was it necessary to carry out the cardiac catheterisation?

65 i. This woman's left atrial and right atrial pressures are essentially equal and there is a step-up in oxygen saturation in the low right atrium. The right heart pressures are abnormally high, as is the left ventricular end-diastolic pressure (for normal ranges of cardiac catheterisation pressures, see Appendix). The woman has an atrial septal defect with mitral regurgitation and tricuspid regurgitation. The association suggests that the septal defect is probably of the ostium primum type (partial atrioventricular canal defect).
ii. The ECG should show (classically) left axis deviation and right bundle branch block.
iii. Catheterisation was traditional to obtain arterial and venous oxygen saturations and to gain further information on any associated lesions. However, echocardiography with Doppler enables calculation of the shunt ratio by using the continuity equation to calculate flow through the mitral and tricuspid valves. It is superior to angiocardiography for showing details of the anatomy. Right ventricular pressure can be calculated from the tricuspid valve regurgitant velocity.

66 i. There has been restenosis of the previously angioplastied lesion.
ii. The overall rate of restenosis after percutaneous transluminal coronary angioplasty (PTCA) is between about 25 and 40%. (In general, the restenosis rate for a PTCA itself performed because of an earlier restenosis is not different from the risk in the initial procedure.) Platelet aggregation and organisation of thrombus (in response to exposure to underlying collagen by the action of the PTCA balloon), vascular recoil, and fibro-intimal (smooth muscle) proliferation have all been implicated in restenosis after angioplasty; as yet no particular agent has been shown to lower the restenosis rate.
iii. The illustration shows that in this patient a coronary stent has been positioned at the site of the previous restenosis. In general, stents have made a substantial impact on the problem of abrupt vessel closure and are the only agents to have made any difference to the longer term restenosis rate. The device used in this case is a Medtronic Wiktor stent, which is made from tantalum and is radio-opaque.

67 A 50-year-old man sustained an anterior myocardial infarction 4 days previously. Since he was admitted 13 hours after the onset of chest pain, thrombolytic therapy was not administered. A nurse noted 'a lot of bruising' on his legs and a test was performed (right). What has happened? (INR, international normalised ratio; APTT, activated partial thromboplastin time, in seconds.)

Haemoglobin	10.9 g/dl
Platelets	34 x 10^9/l
INR	1.9
APTT	64 s (control, 38 s)

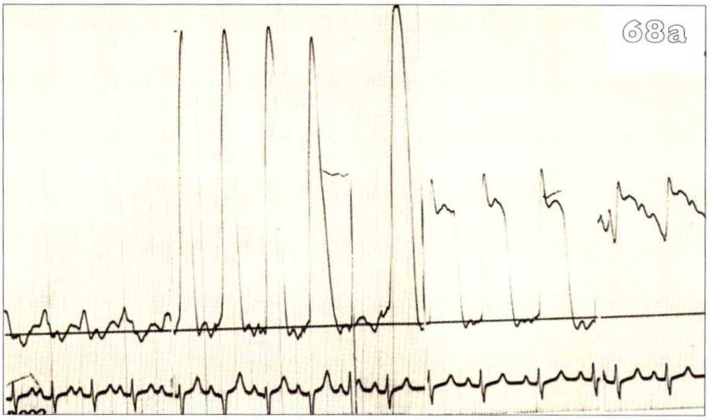

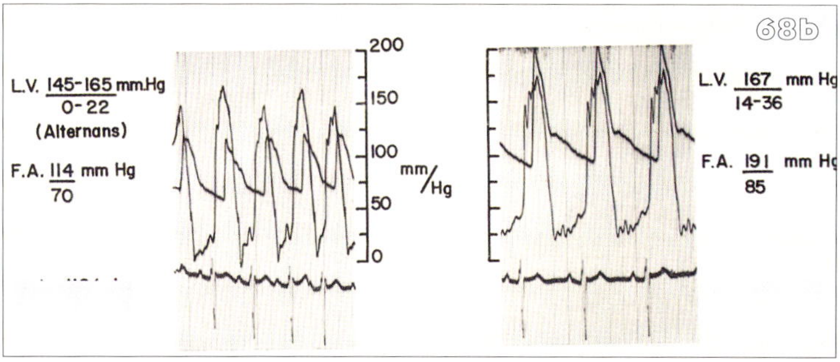

68 The traces shown were obtained at catheterisation of a 35-year-old woman with a late systolic murmur whose elder brother had died suddenly at the age of 38. (LV, left ventricle; FA, femoral artery.)

i. What does **68a** show?

ii. Explain the pharmacological intervention (**68b**).

67 The reduced platelet count, prolonged prothrombin time and increased fibrin degradation products (FDPs) all suggest that disseminated intravascular coagulation (DIC) has developed. The latter is an uncommon, but recognised, complication of myocardial infarction. It follows on from release into the circulation of thromboplastic substances which activate the extrinsic clotting cascade. There follows extensive fibrin formation, followed by fibrin deposition in the microcirculation and massive secondary fibrinolysis. Coagulation factors and platelets are consumed and diffuse haemorrhage can ensue from potential or actual bleeding points. At the same time, there is often thrombosis of peripheral vessels. Despite the fact that the myocardial infarction alone is an adequate cause, other triggers of DIC, such as infection, should be sought and treated. Plasma and platelet infusions are of benefit in patients with diffuse bleeding; in those patients with microcirculatory thrombosis heparin is indicated.

68 **i.** The trace **68a** shows that the left ventricular pressure falls suddenly as the catheter is drawn into the left ventricular outflow tract (Brockenbrough phenomenon). The point at which the pressure falls is subaortic, i.e. neither at the aortic valve itself (aortic stenosis) nor caused by a subvalvar membrane (subvalvar aortic stenosis). This is due to local myocardial hypertrophy and abnormal systolic anterior motion of the mitral valve leaflets. The underlying diagnosis is hypertrophic cardiomyopathy (also known as idiopathic hypertrophic subaortic stenosis, see **3**).
ii. The gradient between the pressure in the main left ventricular chamber and the outflow tract and ascending aorta is reduced during the infusion of phenylephrine (**68b**). The infusion of phenylephrine, a sympathomimetic, produces α-adrenergic peripheral vasoconstriction, which increases afterload on the heart. The increase in resistance to blood flow out of the heart means the left ventricular end-systolic volume is increased and the intraventricular gradient is thereby reduced or abolished. Conversely, inhalation of amyl nitrate (a vasodilator) would lower the afterload and increase the gradient.

69 An unconscious 50-year-old drunk was reviewed in the emergency ward and the ECG shown obtained.
i. Does the man need pacing as an emergency?
ii. What would you do?

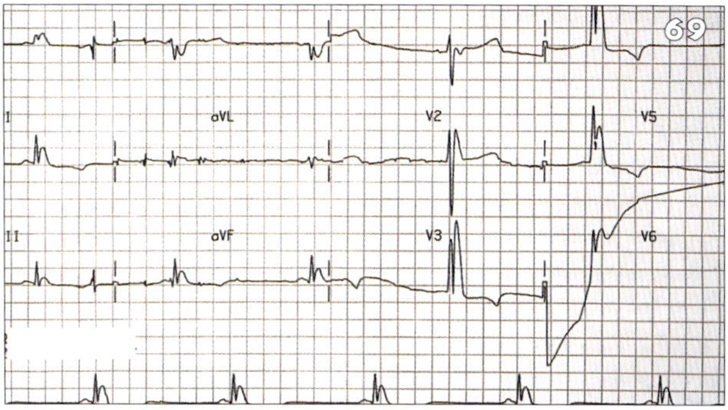

70 This is a coronary artery.
i. Which coronary artery is it?
ii. Name the main branches of this artery.

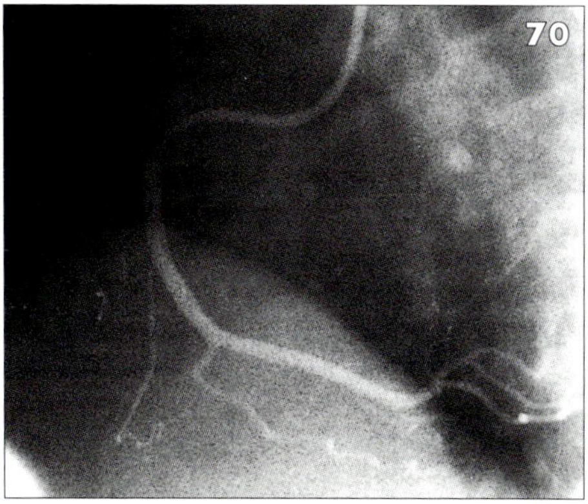

71 The following results were obtained at cardiac catheterisation of a 2-year-old child who had finger clubbing, cyanosis, and failure to thrive.

Chamber	*Pressure (mmHg)*	*O_2 saturation (%)*
SVC	–	43
RA	10 (mean)	42
RV	120/10	43
PA	15/5	42
PCWP	14	96
LA	10	93
LV	120/8	86
Femoral artery	120/8	85

i. List the abnormalities present.
ii. What is the diagnosis?

69 **i.** The ECG is typical of hypothermia. There is: (a) sinus bradycardia, probably due to depression of sinus node activity; (b) obvious J waves, which are narrow convex waves superimposed on the later part of the QRS complex, and are possibly due to early repolarisation; (c) PR and QT prolongation; and artefactual muscular tremor waves due to shivering. With appropriate management (see **ii** below) the heart rate will gradually rise back to normal and electrical pacing will not be necessary.
ii. A rectal temperature should be obtained using a low-reading thermometer. Patients with temperatures between 32–35°C can be restored to normothermia by passive warming only (e.g. by the use of a space blanket or extra clothes). Alcohol (a peripheral vasodilator) promotes heat loss and hypoglycaemia. A temperature below 32°C is often associated with clouding of consciousness or coma and is a medical emergency. Direct surface heat and a space blanket is indicated, as well as the use of warmed intravenous fluids administered slowly. (If hypothyroidism is suspected or confirmed, tri-iodothyronine is given intravenously.) Intensive-care monitoring should be maintained, with careful attention to fluid and electrolyte balance.

70 **i.** The arteriogram demonstrates the right coronary.
ii. The artery runs in the right atrioventricular groove to the posterior aspect of the heart. It supplies the conus artery, the right ventricular or acute marginal branch, the atrioventricular node branch in 60% of individuals, the posterior descending artery in 80% of individuals and the posterior ventricular branches. The posterior descending artery supplies the posterior part of the interventricular septum and the posterior left ventricular wall. In almost 90% of cases, the sinoatrial node is supplied by the right coronary artery.

71 **i.** The right ventricular pressure is grossly elevated; there is a step down in saturation in the left ventricle suggesting a right-to-left shunt of blood from the right ventricle to the left ventricle; and there is a step down in the pressure across the pulmonary valve with a calculated gradient of 105 mmHg across it, indicating severe pulmonary stenosis.
ii. The diagnosis is ventricular septal defect with a right-to-left shunt and pulmonary stenosis. This may form part of Fallot's tetralogy, which is the most common cyanotic congenital heart disease to present after the age of 1 year. It comprises pulmonary stenosis, ventricular septal defect, right ventricular hypertrophy, and overriding of the aorta.

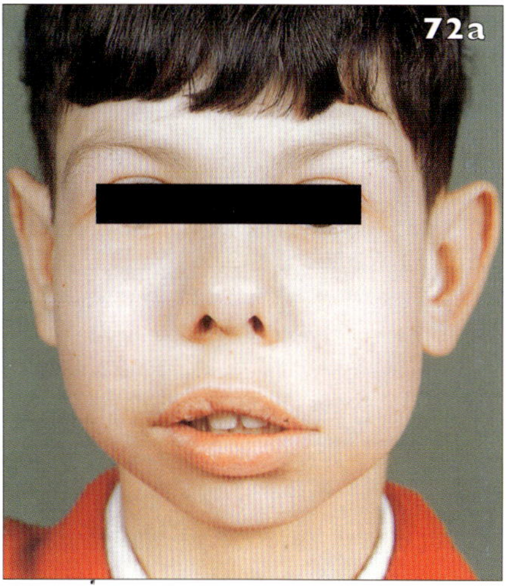

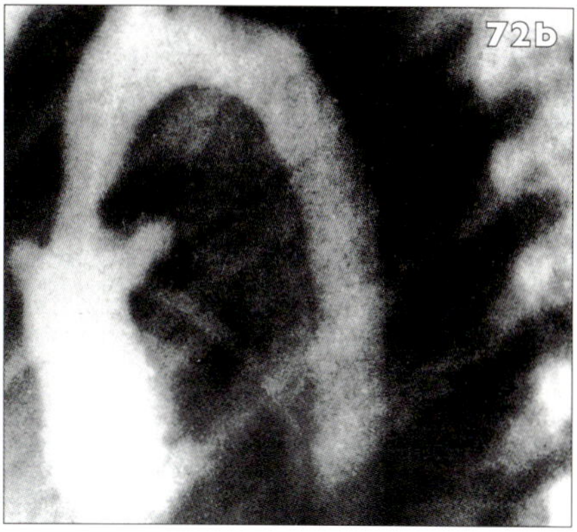

72 **i.** What is the diagnosis?
ii. What is its form of inheritance?
iii. What cardiac lesions are commonly associated with this syndrome?

73 This 35-year-old woman complained of angina, a problem which developed early in members of her family. What is the underlying diagnosis?

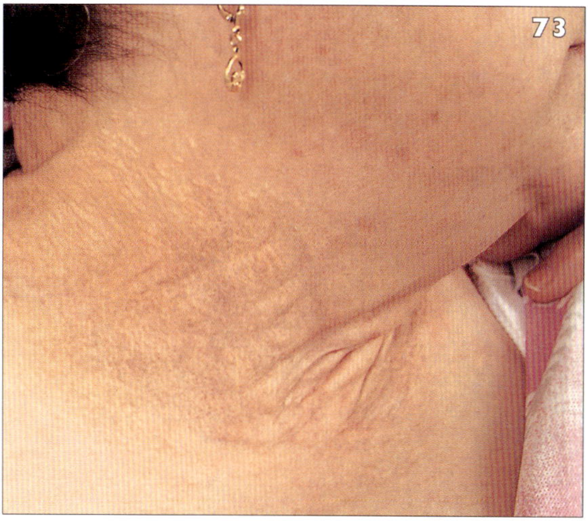

72 **i. 72a** shows a classic 'elfin' facies and **72b** shows an angiogram in which a supravalvar narrowing of the aorta is present. This is Williams' syndrome, which is associated with mental retardation (although with a very positive and extrovert mood), a star-shaped iris, epicanthic folds, strabismus, flattening of the zygoma, low-set ears, thickness of the lips, and infantile hypercalcaemia.
ii. The inheritance is autosomal dominant, although its often sporadic presentation points to a significant rate of new mutations. (*NB* Not all patients with supravalvar aortic stenosis have Williams' syndrome.)
iii. Williams' syndrome is also associated with pulmonary artery branch stenoses. The coronary arteries, which arise below the supravalvar stenosis, are often tortuous and dilated because of the high pressures to which they are subjected. Thoracic aortic aneurysms are also more common, as are other arterial stenoses and irregularities.

73 The skin of the neck shows pseudoxanthoma elasticum. This is an hereditary disorder of elastic tissue (hence the family history of early onset angina pectoris), but the pattern of inheritance and the clinical manifestations are very variable. Pseudoxanthoma elasticum can affect the heart in several ways, most significant of which is an increase in coronary artery disease and myocardial infarction. Mitral valve prolapse is also significantly more common in this group of patients, as is fibro-elastosis of the endocardium. A diffuse pattern of arteriosclerosis of both elastic and muscular arteries develops, akin to that in Mönckeberg's sclerosis. One effect of this can be the complete loss of the radial and ulnar arterial pulses. Non-cardiac features include the 'plucked-chicken' appearance of the skin (shown), gastrointestinal haemorrhage and angioid streaks on funduscopy, due to splits in Bruch's membrane.

74 A 56-year-old man presented with a 6-month history of increasing fatigue and breathlessness. The physical examination revealed a pulse of 80 b.p.m., blood pressure of 120/70 mmHg, venous pressure raised 7 cm, and normal S1 and S2 without an S3. Basal crepitations could also be heard.
i. What is the diagnosis?
ii. What treatment options are there?
iii. Should his children be concerned about inheritance of this condition?

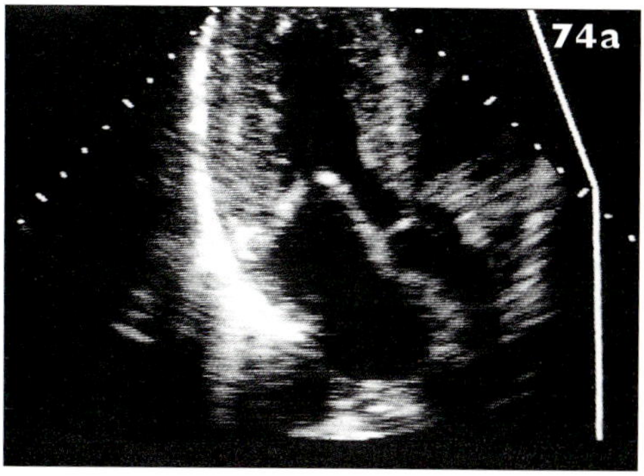
74a

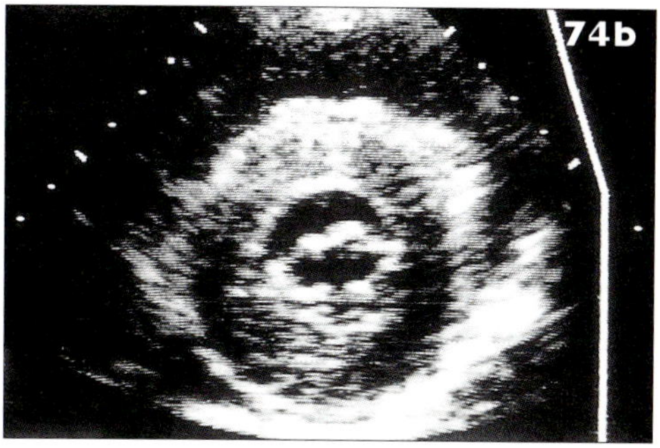
74b

75 A 55-year-old male patient with worsening breathlessness underwent cardiac catheterisation; the table shows the pressures measured.

Chamber	*Pressure (mmHg)*
Pulmonary capillary wedge (mean)	27
Pulmonary artery	45/25
Right ventricle	45/13
Right atrium	a, 10; v, 14
Left ventricle	140/30
Aorta	138/70

i. What is the diagnosis?
ii. What treatment would you recommend?
iii. What is this man's outlook?

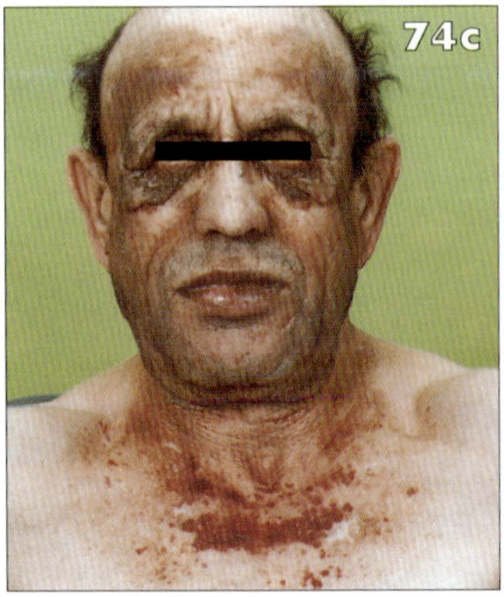

74 **i.** The diagnosis is AL amyloidosis (i.e. primary or idiopathic amyloidosis). The appearance of the patient in **74c** is characteristic of the condition, as in the echocardiograms. Deposition of the inert amyloid fibrils occurs extracellularly within the heart, especially subendocardially and in the conducting tissues. This produces a stiff ventricle with impaired diastolic relaxation. The amyloid deposits appear as extra bright echogenic points in the ventricle.
ii. The treatment options are, unfortunately, very limited. There is no specific treatment and, although necessary for the management of the heart failure, the use of standard drugs is attended by risk. In the case of diuretics, catastrophic volume depletion can occur and digoxin can produce heart block, since the amyloid fibrils bind the drug. Cardiac transplantation is the only definitive therapy.
iii. The majority of cases of *de novo* amyloidosis occur spontaneously. However, several rare hereditary forms of the disease exist, for which specific molecular genetic abnormalities are being defined. Genetic analysis of patients and their close relatives will become increasingly available in the next few years. Considering the age of the patient, the amyloidosis is unlikely to be genetic and may be associated with an occult myeloma.

75 **i.** Analysis of the catheter data shows the pulmonary capillary wedge pressure (and by inference left atrial pressure) to be raised. Pulmonary artery pressure is also raised, as is the right ventricular pressure. The left ventricular systolic pressure is normal, but the end-diastolic pressure is elevated. The left ventricular end-diastolic pressure and the pulmonary artery wedge pressure are about the same. The patient has mitral regurgitation. The right atrial pressure is mildly elevated and the v wave approximates to the right ventricular end-diastolic pressure; tricuspid regurgitation is therefore also present. There is no significant gradient across the aortic valve and the systemic arterial pulse pressure is normal. The diagnosis is mitral and tricuspid regurgitation. (For normal values, see *Appendix 1.*)
ii. In general, the better the left ventricular function, the lower the surgical morbidity and mortality. Valve repair is preferred if possible (in non-rheumatic cases); otherwise valve replacement should be undertaken.
iii. If cases of mitral regurgitation are symptomatic, a degree of impairment of ventricular function is usually already present. This contributes to the overall 5–10% operative mortality of valve replacement. Surgery is therefore timed to be early enough to reduce operative risk and to achieve the best long-term result, but not too early because of the mortality and morbidity of valve replacement and the need for anticoagulant treatment. In non-rheumatic cases with valves suitable for repair, surgery can be carried out much earlier at low risk and with excellent long-term results, including maintenance of sinus rhythm.

76 A 67-year-old woman with worsening but stable angina pectoris on exertion was being assessed with a view to coronary artery bypass surgery. A meticulous young doctor noted a carotid bruit on the left of the neck and ordered a number of investigations, one of which is shown.
i. What is the investigation?
ii. What does it show?
iii. What are the implications for cardiac surgery?

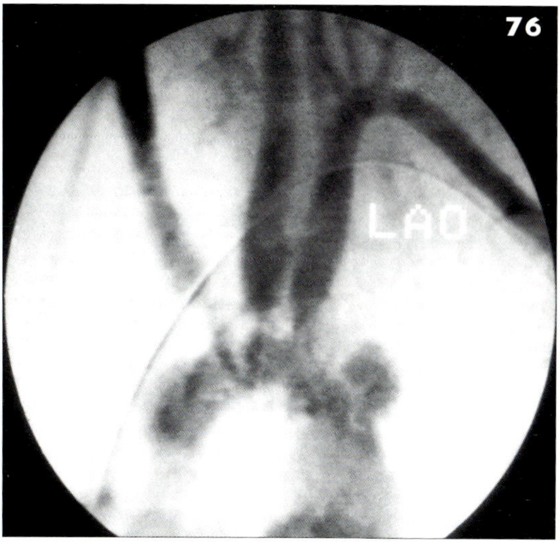

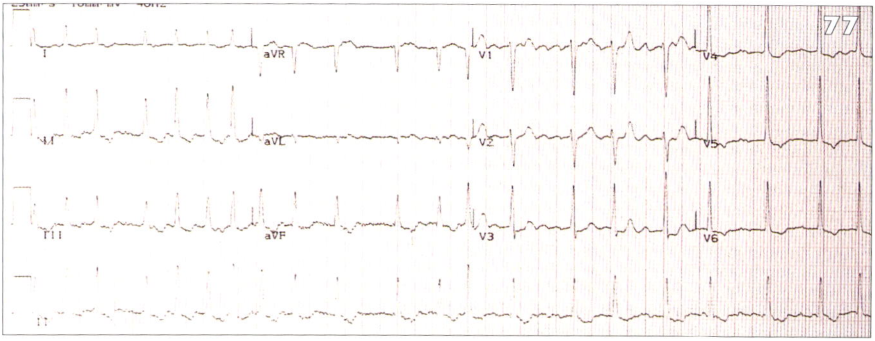

77 A 60-year-old man, known to have had this cardiac rhythm for at least 8 months, had undergone detailed investigations (plasma electrolytes, liver function tests, thyroid function tests, echocardiography and exercise electrocardiography), all of which were essentially normal. He wants you to 'sort the thing out once and for all'.
i. What is the rhythm?
ii. What is the underlying problem?
iii. What are the prognostic implications?
iv. How are you going to 'sort the thing out once and for all'?

76 i. The investigation shown is a digital subtraction angiogram of the carotid arteries.
ii. It shows a significant stenosis in the left common carotid artery.
iii. Whether the carotid stenosis requires surgical attention is a controversial issue. If it is tight (>70%) and symptomatic, carotid endarterectomy is clearly indicated. If it is asymptomatic but the contralateral carotid artery is occluded, many would operate, although the results of a formal trial are still required to clarify the issue. Traditionally, carotid surgery would be performed first as a separate procedure, although combined carotid artery and coronary artery surgery is being undertaken, particularly if the patient has unstable angina. If it is decided to leave an asymptomatic carotid stenosis alone and to perform coronary artery bypass grafting, the increased risk is small (a few percent) and minimised by maintaining pulsatile blood flow during the cardiopulmonary bypass with high perfusion pressure levels. Symptomatic untreated carotid disease increases the morbidity and mortality of the cardiac surgery (up to 25% and 10%, respectively) and should be dealt with by endarterectomy.

77 i. On the ECG there is an absence of P waves and the ventricular rhythm is irregularly irregular, i.e. the patient is in atrial fibrillation (AF).
ii. Virtually all the potential prime causes of atrial fibrillation (e.g. thyroid disease, valve disease, electrolyte disturbances, and alcoholism) have been excluded. In addition, AF is only very rarely a presenting feature of ischaemic heart disease and both the exercise electrocardiography and echocardiogram were normal. By definition, this is a case of 'lone' atrial fibrillation.
iii. There are significant prognostic implications of AF with respect to strokes, but not as regards the development of coronary artery disease or cardiac failure. The overall mortality of untreated AF in these circumstances is approximately double that of healthy matched controls. The incidence of stroke is increased five-fold, the rate of occurrence being proportional to the length of time the patient has been in AF.
iv. In this case, the AF is long-standing so cardioversion is unlikely to be successful. Treatment is aimed at prevention of an excessively rapid ventricular response and prophylaxis against systemic embolism. Digoxin remains the principal agent for control of the ventricular response to AF, although verapamil and beta-blockers can be useful adjuncts. Warfarin anticoagulation is of proven benefit in patients over the age of 65.

78 A 51-year-old woman was admitted to hospital with a sudden left hemiparesis. For 1 month she felt listless, had night sweats, and lost 4 kg in weight. Recently, she had been breathless on exertion and could not sleep without three pillows. She had lost consciousness twice and had been seen in the local hospital emergency room with a seizure a few days earlier, but was not admitted. The attending doctor arranged an appointment with the cardiologist, having heard a new and interesting murmur. The patient had been healthy prior to this illness and had never travelled abroad. On examination she was unwell. Her temperature was 37.6°C, there was no clubbing or splinter haemorrhages, she had a tachycardia of 110 b.p.m., and her blood pressure was 90/60 mmHg. The jugular venous pressure was elevated 4 cm above the sternal angle. On cardiovascular examination, the apex was not displaced and there were no heaves or thrills. The heart sounds were normal and there was a mid-diastolic murmur in the mitral area. There were fine inspiratory crackles at both lung bases. Neurological examination demonstrated a left hemiparesis. The speech was intact and fundi normal. There was no nuchal rigidity and Kernig's sign was absent. Investigations were as shown.

Full blood count:	
Hb	10 g/dl
White cells	8 x 10^9/l
Platelets	340 x 10^9/l
Erythrocyte sedimentation rate	90 mm/h
Biochemistry:	
Sodium	135 mmol/l
Potassium	4.1 mmol/l
Urea	7 mmol/l
(BUN	19.6 mg/dl)

Antinuclear factors: not present.
Chest radiograph: slight enlargement of the heart and moderate pulmonary oedema.

i. Give two differential diagnoses.

79 This exercise ECG was obtained from a 38-year-old woman whose coronary arteries were known to be normal. Give four possible reasons for these appearances.

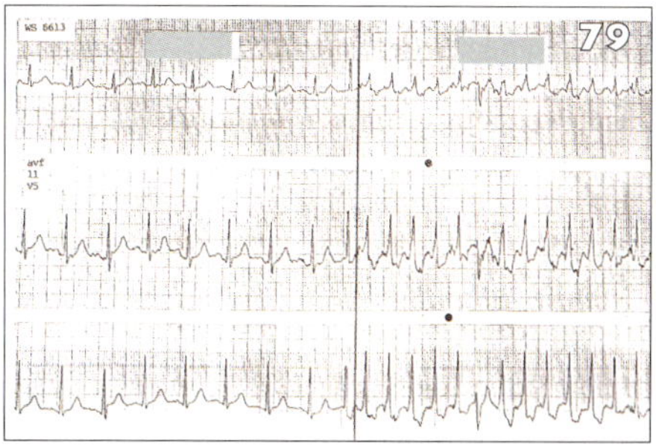

78 **i.** The differential diagnosis is between infective endocarditis affecting a stenosed mitral valve and an atrial myxoma. The former is unlikely for three main reasons – there is no past medical history of rheumatic fever to account for mitral stenosis (congenital mitral stenosis is very rare and would have presented at a younger age); endocarditis is fairly uncommon in mitral stenosis; and it is unusual for the patient not to be in atrial fibrillation in the presence of symptomatic mitral stenosis.
ii. The three most useful tests would be echocardiography, blood cultures, and a CT scan of the brain. An echocardiogram would be most useful in differentiating an atrial myxoma from a vegetation on a stenosed mitral valve. Positive blood cultures would support the diagnosis of endocarditis in this case, if an atrial myxoma was not seen on the echocardiogram. CT scan of the brain would be useful in differentiating an embolic cerebral infarction from an intracerebral haemorrhage. The former can occur with both atrial myxoma and endocarditis, but the latter is more likely to complicate endocarditis and results from a ruptured mycotic aneurysm. Atrial myxoma can present with increasing dyspnoea, systemic emboli, constitutional upset, including a pyrexia of unknown origin, or sudden death. (See also **83**.)

79 This is quite a common clinical scenario, although usually the order of investigations is that the exercise ECG precedes coronary angiography. In the first instance, the resting ECG must be studied. This and other clinical data can aid the exclusion of recognised causes of the 'false positive' exercise test, such as left bundle branch block, digoxin therapy, mitral valve prolapse, Wolf–Parkinson–White syndrome, and left and right ventricular hypertrophy due to whatever cause. In addition, hypokalaemia, hyperventilation, high catecholamine drive and drugs (e.g. tricyclic antidepressants) can all produce confounding ST segment changes. (Anaemia, coronary artery spasm, and aortic stenosis can all produce ischaemic ECG changes, despite angiographically normal coronary arteries; although the exercise test is 'falsely' positive for coronary artery disease, in these cases it is 'truly' positive for ischaemia.)

It is also important to remember that there is a great deal more to the exercise stress tests than just the ECG changes alone; many other features have potential diagnostic or prognostic value, such as reproduction of symptoms (chest pain, dyspnoea, peripheral vasoconstriction, and sweating, fatigue, or dizziness), development of arrhythmias or heart block, failure of heart rate or blood pressure to rise appropriately, and an excessive blood pressure response to exercise.

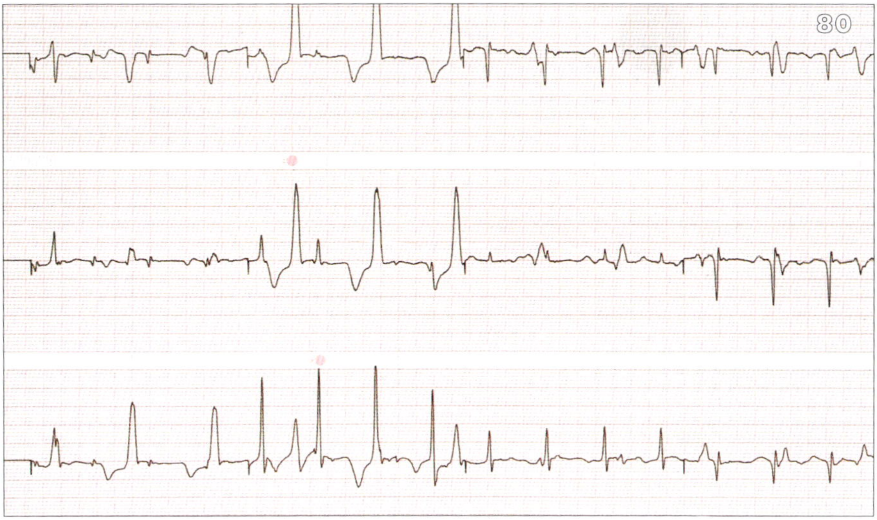

80 This 50-year-old man underwent surgery for end-stage cardiac failure. What was the procedure?

81 A drug derived from this plant (*Digitalis purpurea*) was first used by Withering in the late eighteenth century in the treatment of congestive cardiac failure.

i. What is the drug?

ii. How does it work?

iii. What are the indications for its use?

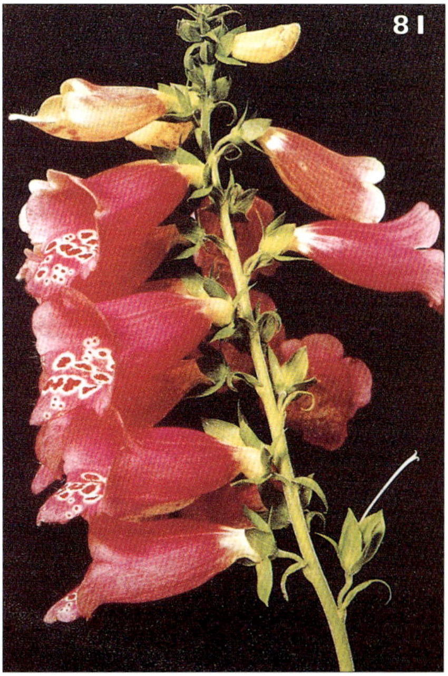

80 This man with end-stage cardiac failure was referred for cardiac transplantation. However, the actual operation performed was not replacement of the recipient heart with a donor organ (orthotopic transplantation), but a 'piggy back' procedure. In this heterotopic transplantation, the donor heart is grafted onto the recipient's circulation in such a manner as to beat and function in parallel with the native heart, the latter not being removed (the ECG shows complexes from both hearts). This procedure is less common than the standard orthotopic replacement. It may offer advantages when the recipient's heart is significantly larger than the donor heart, i.e. where the latter might not be expected to maintain the recipient's circulation on its own. It has also been claimed that the method is of value in patients with increased pulmonary vascular resistance and there is also the (at least theoretical) prospect of the native heart being able to support the circulation during an acute rejection episode in the donor heart. The disadvantages, however, are a higher rate of thromboembolism from the native heart (necessitating anticoagulation) and complex anatomy for the performance of endocardial biopsies.

81 **i.** The plant is the foxglove and the drug is digitalis (in clinical practice, digoxin is the main form used).
ii. The mechanism of action of digitalis is most probably that of inhibition of the cardiomyocyte sarcolemmal Na^+,K^+-ATPase (sodium pump).The transient increase in intracellular sodium produces an accompanying increase in intracellular calcium (via the sodium–calcium exchanger). The increased cytosolic calcium exerts a positive inotropic effect. Parasympathetic activation results in slowing of the sinus node and inhibition of the atrioventricular node. The extent of these effects depends upon the prevailing degree of vagal tone. In addition, weak inhibition of sympathetic nervous activity may be due to a direct effect of digoxin upon sympathetic nerve fibres. In contrast, sympathetic activation, caused by a direct central action of digoxin upon the central nervous system mediated via the μ opiate receptor, is a feature of digoxin toxicity. Thus, the haemodynamic effects of digoxin, at least acutely, are a fall in venous pressure secondary to decreased sympathetic drive; a direct inotropic effect (increased myocardial intracellular calcium), and a reduced heart rate, at least in part vagally mediated. Overall, digoxin is unique in having an inotropic–bradycardiac action, unlike the sympathomimetic inotropes which tend to produce tachycardia with any positive inotropic effect.
iii. The clearest indications for its use is chronic atrial fibrillation, particularly in the context of congestive cardiac failure (CCF). Its use as a mild inotrope in CCF in sinus rhythm has recently increased. However, digoxin has no rate-slowing effect in patients with CCF in sinus rhythm and its usefulness is dependent upon its inotropism. Conversely, its main benefit in atrial fibrillation is slowing of the ventricular rate, which is often the main (or only) cause of the heart failure.

82 A 10-year-old Cuban girl gave a 4-day history of pain in both ankle joints, 2 days after which she developed left inframammary pain that was worse on inspiration and on lying flat. She was admitted to hospital. During the next 48 hours she complained of a painful swelling over the left knee and pain in the right elbow. She had a history of recurrent tonsillitis. On examination she had a temperature of 37.8°C and her throat was clear. Auscultation of the heart revealed a soft pericardial rub and a soft systolic murmur at the apex. The heart sounds were normal and there were no murmurs. The chest was clear. Examination of the locomotor system demonstrated a swollen and tender left ankle with painful, restricted movements. She was also tender over the right ankle and the right elbow joint, but her calves were not swollen or tender. The results of abdominal and neurological examinations were normal. Investigations are shown at the right

i. What is the differential diagnosis?

ii. What is the most probable diagnosis?

Full blood count:

Haemoglobin	11.1 g/dl
White cells	12 x 10^9/l
Platelets	160 x 10^9/l
Erythrocyte sedimentation rate	64 mm/h

Blood cultures (x two): no growth.

Chest and left ankle radiographs: normal.

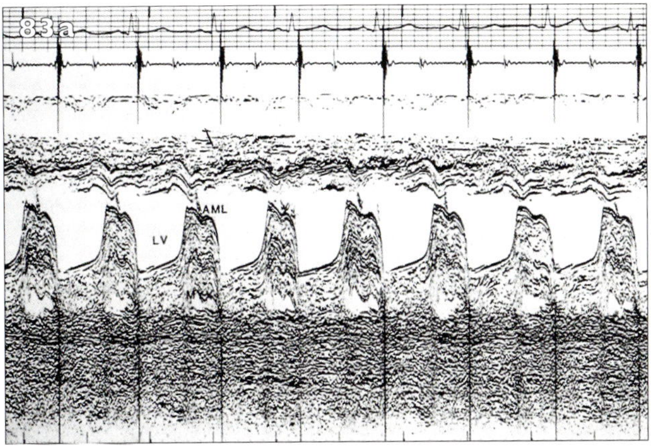

83 This investigation was performed in a patient who had experienced two episodes of sudden loss of consciousness. What is the investigation and what does it show?

82 **i.** The differential diagnoses are rheumatic fever, systemic lupus erythematosis, acute juvenile arthritis, infective endocarditis, or a viral illness causing arthritis and pericarditis.
ii. The most probable diagnosis is rheumatic fever. The clue comes from the history of recurrent tonsillitis, which is suggestive of probable previous beta-haemolytic streptococcal infection. The diagnosis of rheumatic fever is usually made on clinical grounds. There are no specific tests to diagnose the condition. The Duckett–Jones criteria for diagnosing rheumatic fever have been used for over half a century (see **13**). In this case the arthritis and carditis form the two major criteria. She has a fever, arthralgia and a raised ESR, which are all minor criteria. Raised anti-streptolysin O (ASO) titres would lend further support to previous streptococcal infection. It would be prudent to exclude other conditions which can present in this way. An echocardiogram would be useful to check for vegetations and to exclude a pericardial effusion. Aspiration of the knee joint followed by microscopy and culture would be necessary to exclude a streptococcal arthritis, although in such cases the blood cultures are almost always positive unless the patient has had prior antibiotics. A full autoimmune screen should also be performed to exclude connective tissue disease.

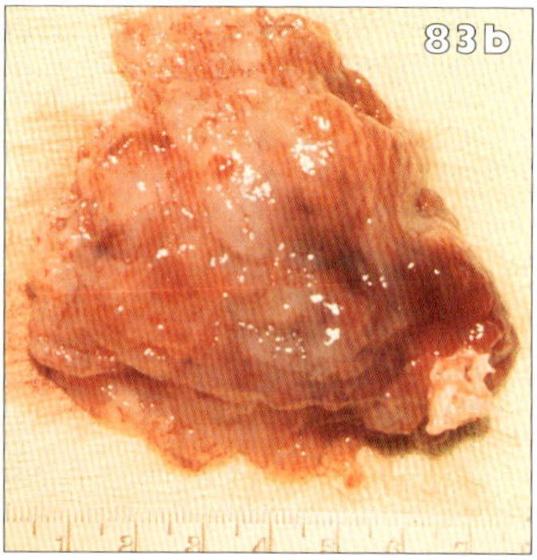
83b

83 The M mode echocardiographic study (**83a**) shows a mass – a myxoma – in the left atrium. It shows a 'filling in' of the mitral valve orifice during diastole. There is a slight delay between the opening of the mitral valve leaflets and the echoes appearing between the leaflets. This delay corresponds to the time taken for the tumour to travel from the left atrium to the mitral valve orifice. On a 2D image the mass may be identified as arising from the atrial septum. Myxomata (**83b**) are the most common primary tumours of the heart, three-quarters of them being found in the left atrium. They are typically pedunculated and attached to the fossa ovalis, highly mobile, and prolapse forwards during diastole. This behaviour produces haemodynamic effects akin to an atrial ball-valve thrombus and patients may present with syncope or breathlessness. Clinically, the abrupt halt of the forwards movement of the myxoma can be heard as a mid-diastolic murmur and a 'tumour plop', which sounds like a late opening snap. These tumours give rise to systemic symptoms such as fever and, because the gelatinous masses are often very friable, embolisation is common. Haemolysis may occur. (*NB* The features of left atrial myxoma which distinguish it clinically from mitral stenosis are classically the variability of the auscultatory features – although the 'plop' sounds like an opening snap it occurs later; in addition the mid-diastolic murmur of atrial myxoma is shorter than the diastolic murmur of mitral stenosis, since flow stops when the myxoma engages the mitral valve. Also, atrial fibrillation is rare in myxoma.)

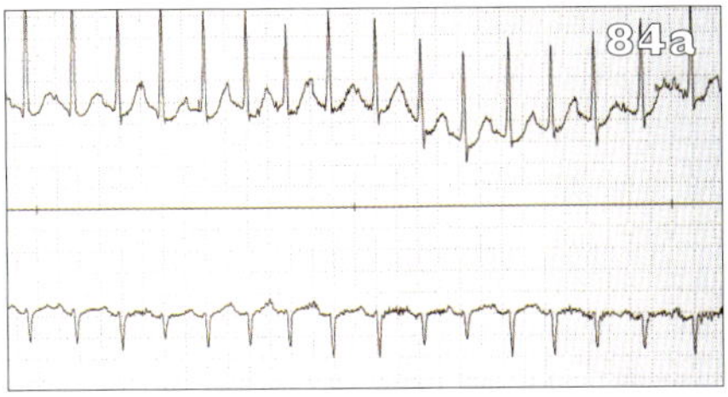

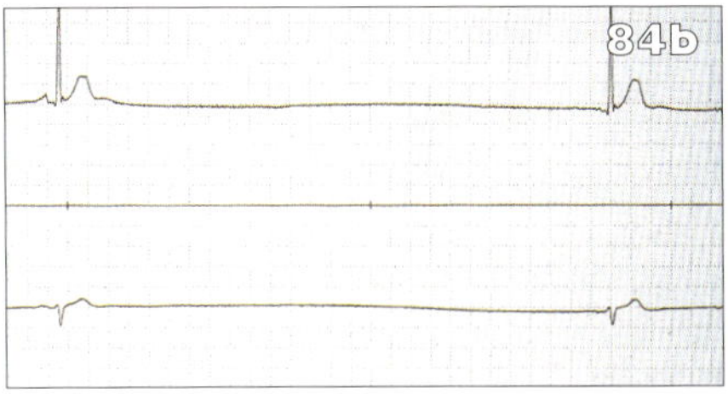

84 A 70-year-old man complaining of 'feeling giddy' underwent an investigation, the results of which are shown.
i. What was the investigation?
ii. What abnormalities did it display?
iii. How would you manage the patient?

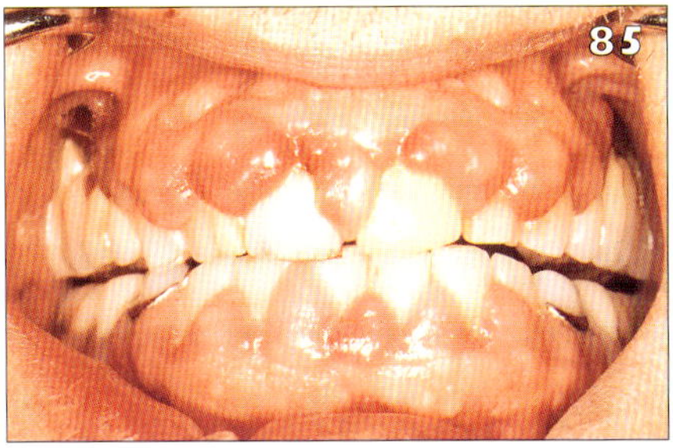

85 This patient with primary pulmonary hypertension has been receiving intensive medical treatment for several months.
i. What is shown?
ii. What is the likely cause?
iii. Suggest another agent that can cause the effect noted in **i**?

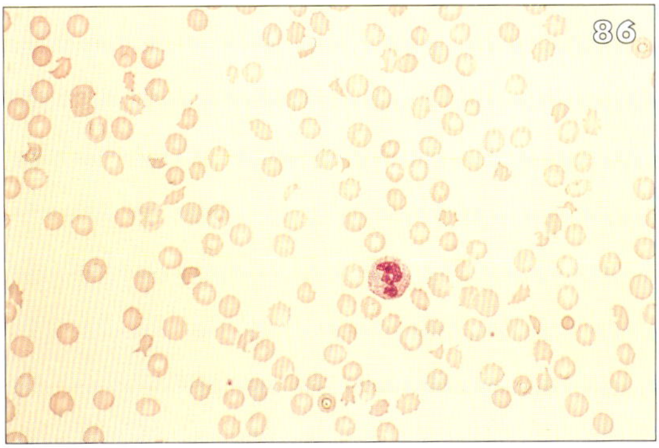

86 This is a blood film from a 70-year-old woman with a Starr–Edwards aortic valve prosthesis who presented with breathlessness. She was apyrexial and had a loud opening click, a soft systolic murmur in the aortic area followed by a loud prosthetic component to the second heart sound, and an early diastolic murmur. Her haemoglobin was 6.1 g/dl, a chest radiograph demonstrated a slightly enlarged heart, but the lung fields were clear.
i. What are the abnormal findings on the blood film?
ii. What is the cause of her anaemia and which further tests would you perform to confirm this?

84 **i.** A 24-hour ambulatory ECG (Holter) was performed.
ii. There are episodes of supraventricular tachycardia as well as periods of profound bradycardia. This is the 'sick sinus' or 'tachy–brady' syndrome. The 'giddiness' comprised palpitations due to supraventricular tachycardia (SVT, **84a**) and presyncope due to long sinus pauses (**84b**).
iii. A number of different pathophysiological processes can lead to the sick sinus syndrome. The exact nature of the dysfunction of the sinus node is the central issue, e.g. whether an essentially healthy sinus node is affected by abnormal autonomic inputs, or whether the nodal tissues are diseased. In the latter case, there can be extensive destruction of the atrial automatic tissues with inflammation, fibrosis, and degeneration of the associated nerves and ganglia. This can occur with remarkably little disease elsewhere in the heart or coronary circulation. As well as the bradycardia, paroxysms of regular and/or irregular atrial tachyarrhythmias frequently occur, constituting the 'tachy' component of the 'tachy–brady' syndrome. As far as treatment is concerned, the patient will need a permanent pacing system inserted, with drug therapy for the tachycardia. [NB: Drug therapy for SVT without pacing (for example b-blockade or digoxin for paroxysmal atrial fibrillation) can worsen sinus node function even further. Since the patient is otherwise fit and the pauses are due to sinus node dysfunction, an atrial pacing system would suffice.]

85 **i.** Gross gum hypertrophy is shown.
ii. The most likely cause is the use of high doses of nifedipine. Although the current management of primary pulmonary hypertension is suboptimal, calcium antagonists have shown some promise in milder cases. Nifedipine has been shown to improve New York Heart Association functional class, as well as electrocardiographic characteristics (QRS axis and R wave height in V1) and echocardiographic parameters (right ventricular internal dimension with M mode). (These indices of function can measure the chronic effects of therapy; earlier studies emphasised acute changes in pulmonary arterial pressure and pulmonary vascular resistance.)
iii. The most commonly used cardiological drug that causes gum hypertrophy is cyclosporin, the use of which in immunosuppression has transformed the outlook of cardiac transplantation patients.

86 **i.** The blood film reveals red cell fragmentation and anisocytosis. These are features of a microangiopathic haemolytic anaemia.
ii. The anaemia is due to mechanical red cell haemolysis caused by the prosthetic valve and the paravalvar leak. This can be confirmed by finding an increase in reticulocytes, a reduction in serum haptoglobin levels and raised urinary haemosiderin levels. In this case, the prosthetic aortic valve requires further assessment. It is prudent to exclude prosthetic valve endocarditis, because this can lead to valve malfunction with concomitant valve haemolysis. Mild haemolysis with mechanical prosthetic valves is not unusual and can lead to iron-deficiency anaemia in the long term. This is easily managed with iron supplements.

87 This phonocardiogram was obtained from a university student who complained of chest pain which commenced in her second term of studies.
i. What are the features labelled A to C?
ii. What is the diagnosis?
iii. Relate two clinical phenomena associated with this condition.

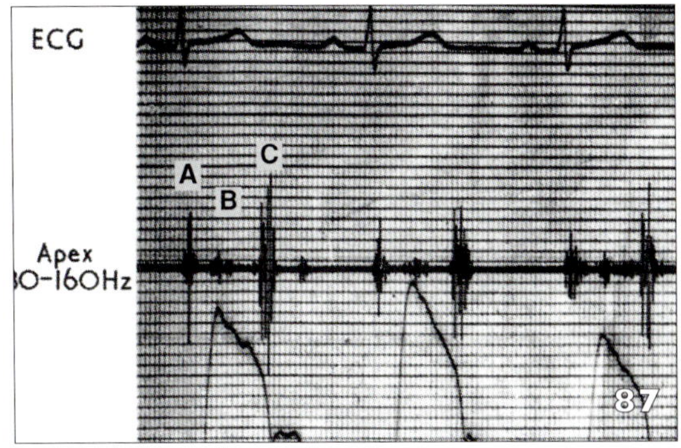

88 Can you relate (**88a**) and (**88b**), clinically and pathophysiologically?

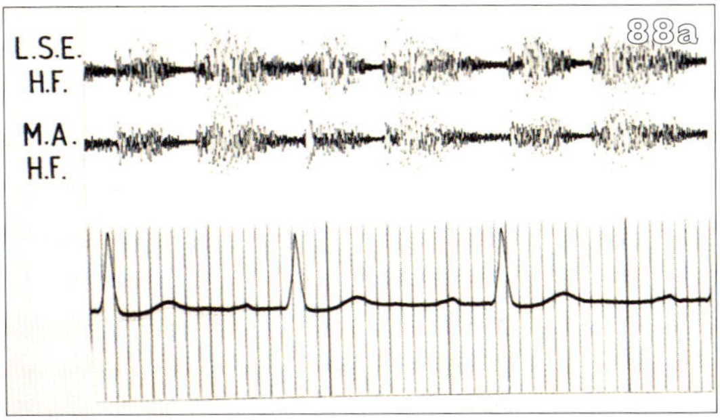

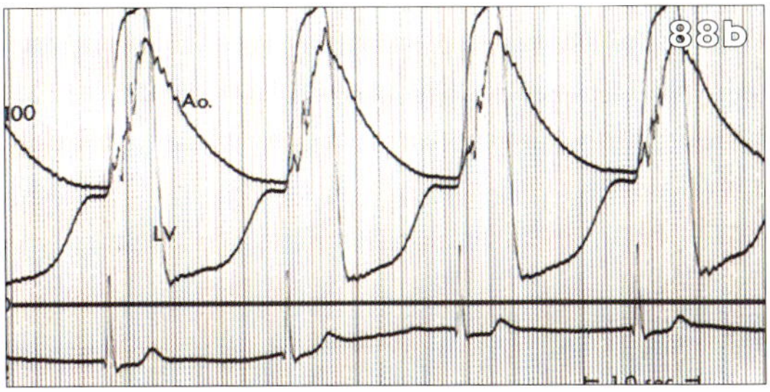

87 **i.** A, the first heart sound; B, mid-systolic click; C, the second heart sound.
ii. The diagnosis is mitral valve prolapse.
iii. Prolapse of the mitral valve leaflets into the left atrium occurs when the left ventricular chamber size is at its smallest, i.e. late systole. It is more likely to occur in conditions in which the valve leaflets are enlarged with redundant tissue (floppy mitral valve) or where there is weakening or stretching of the subvalvar apparatus. Secondary mitral valve prolapse (which can carry a poor prognosis) must be distinguished from primary mitral valve prolapse, which is essentially benign. This young woman has symptoms of the 'mitral valve prolapse syndrome'. A late systolic murmur would indicate a measure of mitral regurgitation, and such a patient should receive antibiotic prophylaxis for endocarditis. Clinical features of the syndrome include palpitations (mainly ventricular ectopic beats during exercise), atypical chest pain, dizziness and an increased incidence of panic disorder. Stroke is a rare complication that has been reported, perhaps due to embolism of platelet thrombus formed in the angle between the prolapsing leaflet and the left atrial wall. Most patients with floppy mitral valves are asymptomatic. In the mitral valve prolapse syndrome, the symptoms cannot be attributed to the severity of mitral reflux, which is often trivial.

88 The pathophysiological basis of aortic regurgitation is a failure of competent coaptation of the aortic valve leaflets, due to dilatation of the aortic root and stretch of the valve ring (syphilitic or other aortitis or aortic aneurysm); thickening of aortic valve leaflets and adhesions between them which impairs movement of the leaflets back to full apposition (e.g. rheumatic fever); or leaflet perforation (e.g. in infective endocarditis). Incompetence of the aortic valve produces volume loading of the left ventricle which becomes hypertrophied and enlarged. The heart may compensate effectively for this handicap, but if the regurgitation is sufficiently severe, the left ventricle ultimately fails. The auscultatory and haemodynamic consequences are shown in (**88a**) and (**88b**). The phonocardiogram shows a mild mid-systolic flow murmur audible at the left sternal edge (LSE) and an early diastolic murmur, which begins immediately after the second heart sound, is of high frequency (HF), and occupies diastole. The transducer at the mid-axillary location (MA) shows that a mid-diastolic murmur is also detectable at this point (Austin Flint murmur). The pressure trace confirms the above: the arterial pulse pressure is abnormally wide and the left ventricular end-diastolic pressure rises steadily during diastole, virtually to equal the aortic end-diastolic pressure. This is severe aortic regurgitation.

89 A 70-year-old West African man was admitted, through the emergency department, complaining of headache and confusion. After a few minutes, he had a grand mal seizure.
i. Suggest a diagnosis.
ii. What is the treatment?
iii. What is the outlook?

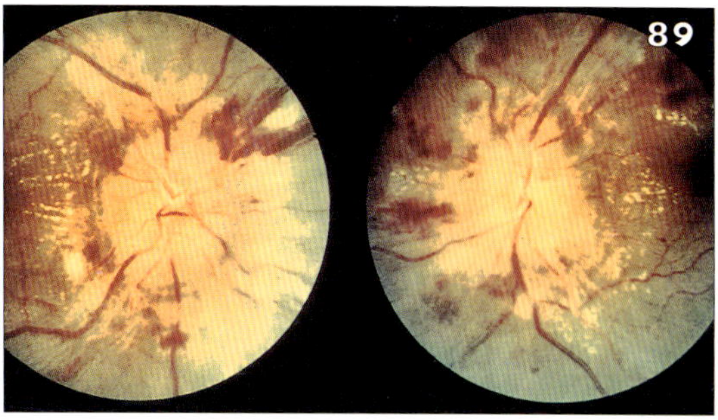
89

90 This is an ECG of a 15-year-old boy who has had a cardiac murmur. On examination, he was found to be cyanosed and had finger clubbing. On examination of the precordium there was a prominent left parasternal heave. The second heart sound was palpable in the pulmonary area. There was a soft systolic murmur in the pulmonary area with a single second heart sound.

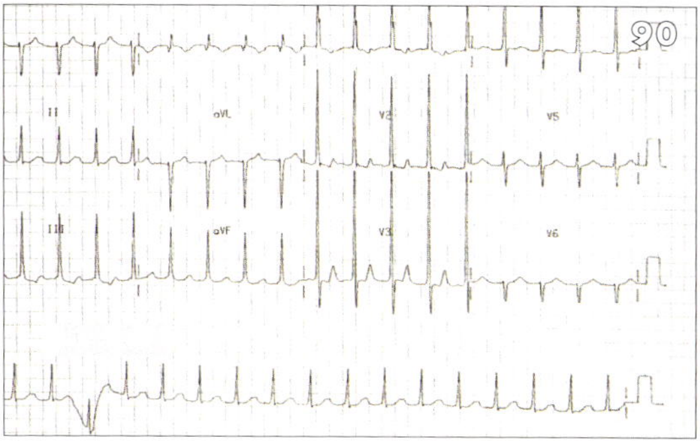

90

i. List three abnormalities on the ECG.
ii. What comment can you make on cardiac chamber sizes from study of the ECG?
iii. What is the probable diagnosis?
iv. What is the management?

91 This hypertensive 27-year-old man was investigated as an out-patient.
i. What abnormalities can be seen on this chest radiograph?
ii. What physical sign do you think might be elicited?
iii. Name the definitive treatment?
iv. What are the long-term complications of **iii**?

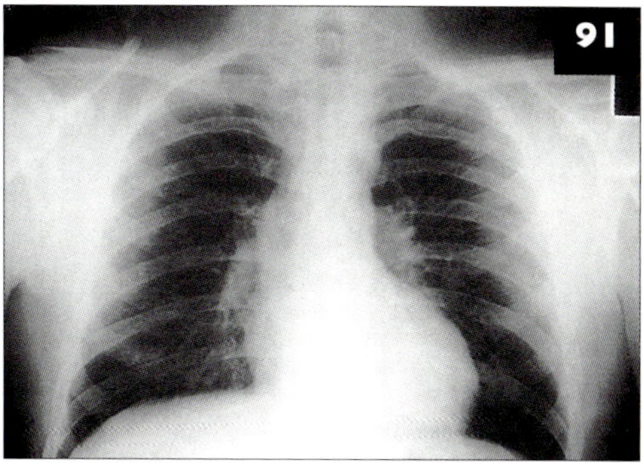
91

89 i. The fundus shows grade IV changes of hypertensive retinopathy. The patient had hypertensive encephalopathy.
ii. This is a medical emergency, but there is a danger of cerebral infarction and blindness if the blood pressure fall is too precipitous. This is of particular relevance in older patients. A wide range of drugs has been used. The combined alpha- and beta-blocker labetalol is safe and effective. Sodium nitroprusside is effective, but requires careful monitoring, with caution for rebound hypertension on withdrawal of the drug. Hydralazine (especially in conjunction with a beta-blocker) is also an effective option. Underlying causes of hypertension must be sought and treatment continued.
iii. Untreated, malignant hypertension is almost inevitably fatal within a few months, due to severe end-organ damage, particularly of the brain, heart and kidney. With effective treatment and no established end-organ damage, the outlook should be excellent.

90 i. Three abnormalities are first-degree atrioventricular block (the PR interval exceeds 220 ms); extreme rightward axis; and voltage criteria consistent with right ventricular hypertrophy.
ii. The right ventricle is hypertrophied.
iii. The most probable diagnosis is a ventricular septal defect with shunt reversal (Eisenmenger's syndrome). Other possibilities include Fallot's tetralogy.
iv. The management should be medical therapy. Ventricular septal defect is the most common congenital heart lesion and accounts for 1/500 live births. Spontaneous closure occurs in nearly 50% of cases, but large defects need to be corrected surgically. If a child is failing to thrive the defect should be closed at about 3 months of age. In children with symptoms controlled by diuretics and digoxin the defect should be closed as soon as possible. If the pulmonary vascular resistance is calculated at above 8 units at cardiac catheterisation, surgery is not usually advised due to the risk of precipitating severe right ventricular failure. Cyanosis at rest in this patient indicates that shunt reversal has already developed due to pulmonary hypertension. In the long term, heart and lung transplantation is the definitive therapeutic option.

91 i. The chest radiograph shows notching of the inferior aspect of the 4th to 8th ribs. This has been caused by pressure from dilated posterior intercostal arteries. The aortic knuckle appears flattened because of the dilated left subclavian artery above, which obscures it. The patient has coarctation of the aorta.
ii. The key physical sign is that of delay between the radial and femoral pulses, a direct mechanical consequence of the arterial stenosis located between the two pulses.
iii. Definitive management requires surgical resection of the coarctation. This should be performed as early as feasible after its discovery. Provided that it is an uncomplicated case, with the arterial duct already closed, resection of the coarcted segment and end-to-end anastomosis should be achievable.
iv. Long-term complications of the surgery include spinal cord injury during the period of aortic clamping and increased hypertension in the early post-operative period; re-coarctation and aneurysm formation (especially if prosthetic patches have been incorporated in the repair) are local complications. Premature coronary artery disease and endocarditis of a bicuspid aortic valve are other late complications which may occur.

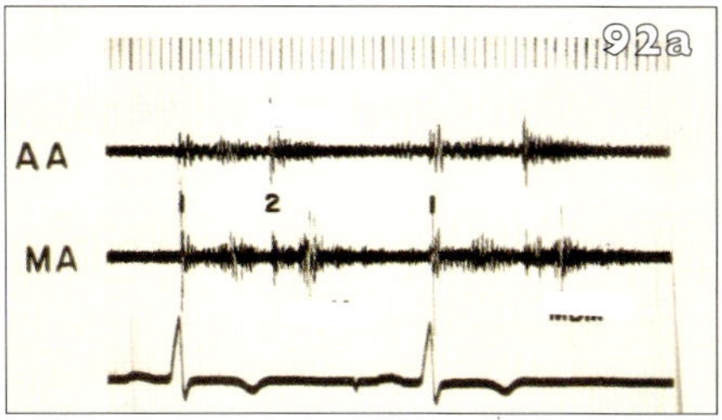

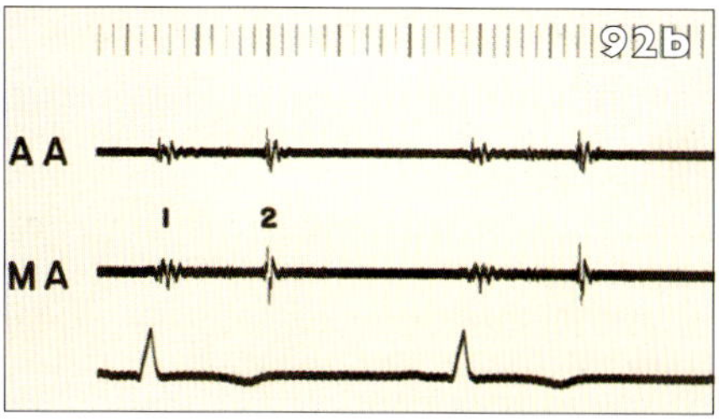

92 A 24-year-old male underwent cardiac surgery. The traces reflect the auscultatory findings before (**92a**) and after (**92b**) the operation (AA, aortic area; MA, mid-axilla). What was the disorder which necessitated the operation?

93 These ECGs were obtained from a patient who had been admitted with a severe episode of central chest pain 1 week previously.
i. What event occurred?
ii. What prognostic information can you obtain from the ECGs?

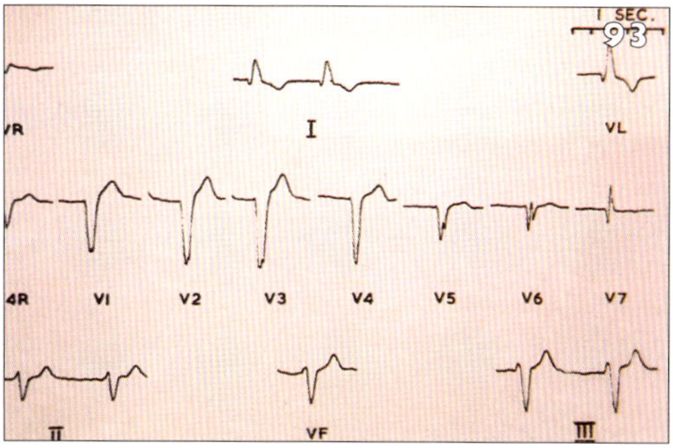

94 A 60-year-old man suffered an anterior myocardial infarction 9 months before this radiograph was taken.
i. What does the radiograph show?
ii. How does this influence prognosis?
iii. What interventions have been shown to prevent this?

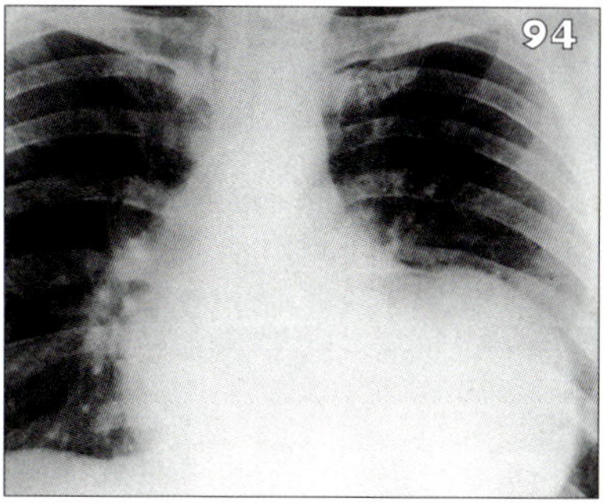

92 In the pre-operative trace (**92a**), the key features are an early diastolic murmur, maximal at the aortic area (AA) and a mid-diastolic murmur audible in the mitral area. As well as these, there is a soft mitral mid-systolic murmur. The heart sounds (S1 and S2) are normal. In the post-operative trace (**92b**), the murmurs have disappeared and S2 is slightly longer and of an altered quality of sound compared to the S2 in the pre-operative trace. The patient had pure aortic regurgitation. The early diastolic murmur is the classic murmur of this condition and commences when the left ventricular pressure falls below that in the aorta and blood regurgitates back into the left ventricle. The mitral mid-diastolic murmur is an Austin Flint murmur, named after the physician who first described it in 1862. The severity of the aortic regurgitation is related neither to the length of the aortic early diastolic murmur nor to the presence, absence, or duration of the Austin Flint murmur. The mechanism of the Austin Flint murmur is oscillation and part closure of the anterior mitral valve leaflet caused by the regurgitant jet striking it.

93 **i.** The patient sustained an anterior myocardial infarction. The typical setting for the left bundle branch block produced would be a proximal left anterior descending coronary artery thrombosis with infarction of the territory supplied by the first septal perforator branch. The latter territory includes the left anterosuperior fascicle.
ii. Anterior infarction complicated by left bundle branch block carries a particularly poor prognosis. This reflects the large territory of heart muscle damaged. Second-degree block (Mobitz Type II) is also common in this presentation of anterior myocardial infarction; sudden progression to complete heart block is a recognised complication.

94 **i.** The radiograph shows a left ventricular aneurysm.
ii. Development of a left ventricular aneurysm indicates a poorer prognosis, both in terms of the larger initial degree of myocardial damage necessary to produce the aneurysm and also the increased likelihood of late ventricular dilatation ('remodelling'). As chamber size gradually increases, congestive cardiac failure develops in at least 20% of such patients. There is also a greater risk of ventricular arrhythmias and of systemic embolisation from mural thrombus.
iii. Generally speaking, late ventricular dilatation is less likely in a myocardial territory subtended by a patent coronary artery rather than an occluded vessel. Thus, revascularisation (either percutaneous transluminal coronary angioplasty or coronary artery bypass grafting) reduce the likelihood of this complication developing. If aneurysm formation has already occurred by the time of bypass surgery, left ventricular aneurysmectomy may normalise the geometry of the left ventricular chamber and improve its mechanical properties. The Survival and Ventricular Enlargement (SAVE) trials suggest that angiotensin-converting enzyme inhibitors are of clear benefit in reducing the morbidity and mortality due to development of heart failure after myocardial infarction.

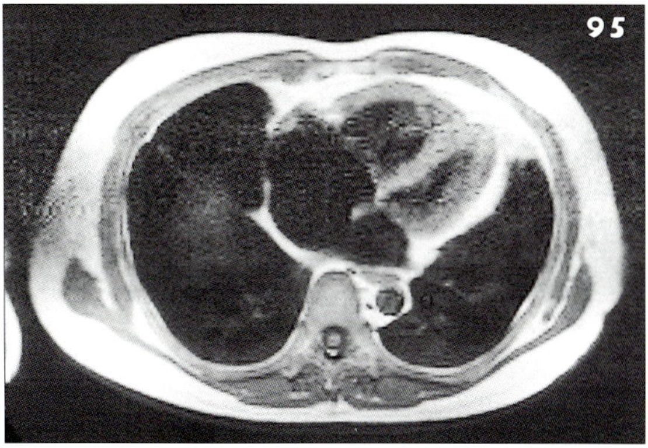
95

95 This image was obtained from an asymptomatic 7-year-old child.

i. What is the diagnosis?

ii. What should be done and what is the prognosis after definitive treatment?

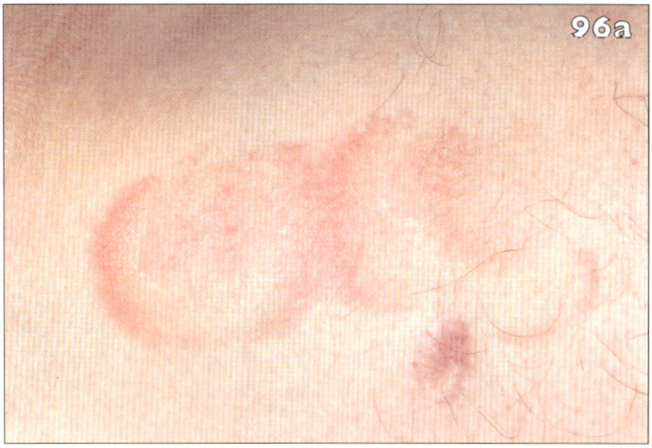
96a

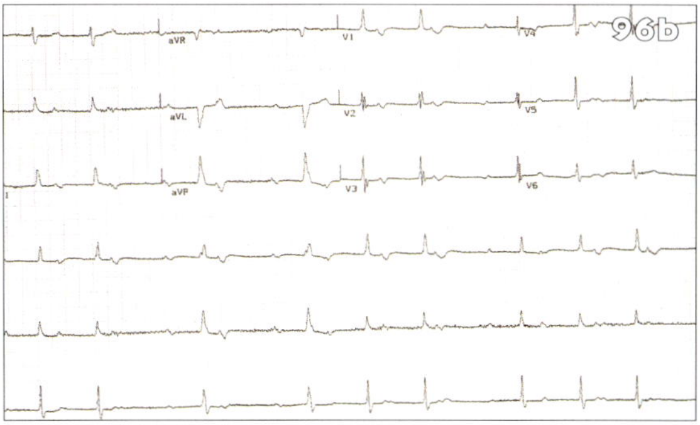

96b

96 A 23-year-old woman returned from a 3-week holiday abroad complaining of lethargy, myalgia, headache and dizziness on exertion. There was no past medical history of note, with the exception of a tender rash which was noted on holiday and attributed to an insect bite. Fortunately, a friend had taken a photograph of this rash (**96a**). On examination she was afebrile, her heart rate was slow, and she had mild nuchal rigidity and a right-sided lower motor neurone seventh nerve palsy. An ECG and rhythm strip taken from the patient is shown in **96b**.

What is the diagnosis and how would you confirm it?

95 i. This spin echo MRI shows an atrial septal defect (ASD) and a dilated right atrium and right ventricle. In addition, the anterior leaflet of the mitral valve attaches to the same point as that to which the septal leaflet of the tricuspid valve attaches. This is an ostium primum atrial septal defect. It is observations such as the latter for which MRI is of particular value in the assessment of ASDs, as well as for measurement of the pulmonary systemic shunt ratio by means of velocity mapping. However, as noted in **22**, MRI is essentially a research technique for clinical problems such as these; echocardiography is at least as good for obtaining the required information.
ii. As in most cases of uncomplicated ASD in childhood, surgical repair should be undertaken reasonably soon after diagnosis. Recently, per catheter methods of closure have been increasingly employed for straightforward secundum defects, in particular using double umbrella devices (e.g. Rashkind duct umbrella) and the Sideris buttoned double-disc device. A coherent rim of atrial septal tissue must surround the ASD, so ostium primum defects do not lend themselves to these techniques of closure. The mortality of formal open surgical repair is low (<1%) and the prognosis is excellent, provided competence of the mitral valve can be achieved. The cleft anterior mitral valve leaflet needs to be repaired.

96 **96a** has the appearance of erythema chronicum migrans. The ECG rhythm in **96b** shows complete heart block. Taken together with the history and the facial nerve palsy the diagnosis is Lyme disease. Lyme disease is a tick-borne disease caused by the spirochete *Borrelia burgdorferi*. In the first stage of the illness there is the appearance of a characteristic skin lesion at the site of the tick bite, which usually begins as a red macule or papule and then expands with partial central clearing. This is known as erythema chronicum migrans. It is associated with regional lymphadenopathy, flu-like symptoms and joint pains. Weeks or months afterwards, the second stage of the disease occurs during which there is a combination of cardiac and neurological involvement. Cardiac manifestations include second or third degree atrioventricular block, pericarditis and mild left ventricular dysfunction. Cardiac involvement is brief, but the manifestations may recur. Meningitis, encephalitis and cranial nerve involvement, particularly seventh nerve palsy, form part of the neurological effects of the disease.

The organism can be isolated from the blood or the cerebrospinal fluid, but the yield is low. IgM antibody specific to the spirochete is present early in the disease. Treatment comprises high dose intravenous penicillin for 10 days. Prednisolone is occasionally prescribed in atrioventricular block.

97 A 60-year-old man was undergoing a number of regular investigations as part of a drug trial, having experienced an acute anterior myocardial infarction 6 weeks previously.
i. What does this investigation show?
ii. What would you do?
iii. What is the natural history?

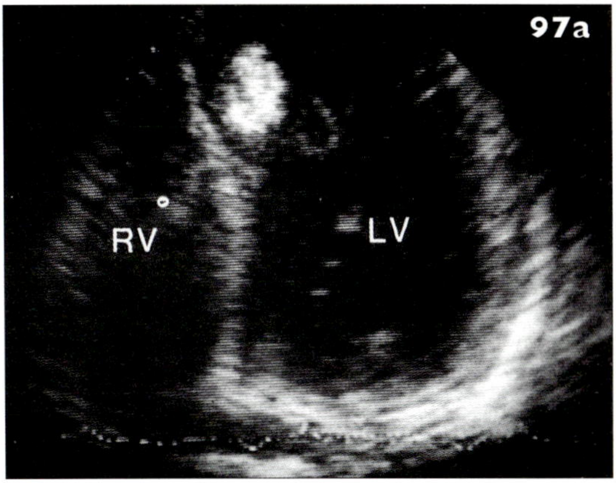

98 A patient on the coronary care unit who had been admitted with a first infarction experienced a 'faint' 18 hours after admission.
i. What does the ECG show?
ii. What is the likely anatomical origin of the disturbance?
iii. How would you treat it?
iv. What if this had occurred four weeks after admission?

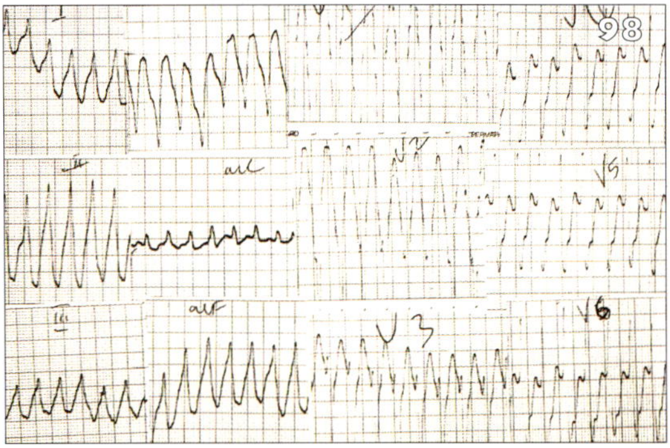

99 What is the abnormality on this chest radiograph?

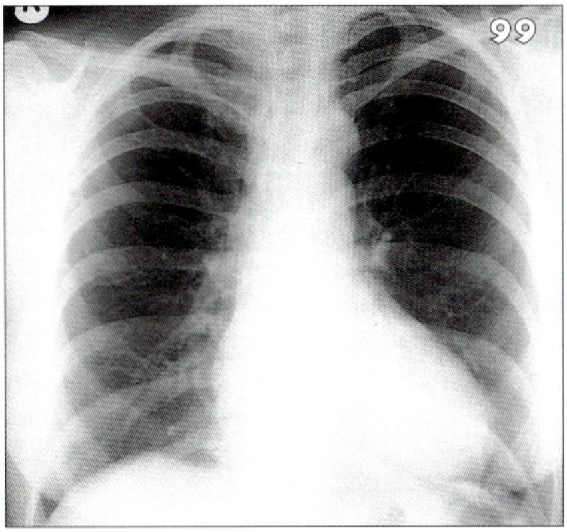

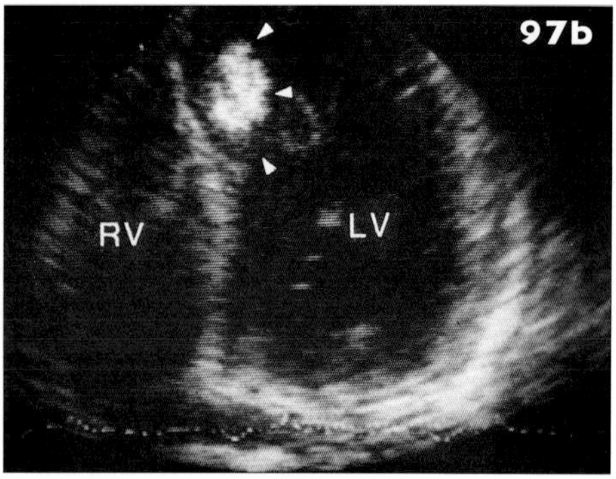

97 **i.** This is a 2D echocardiogram, four-chamber view, showing thrombus at the apex of the left ventricle (arrows).
ii. In the context of this question, the thrombus is probably quite well organised; however, oral anticoagulation does improve the prognosis with respect to the risk of stroke.
iii. The prevalence of this complication of myocardial infarction (MI) is about 45% in patients who die early after MI. About 10% of patients who die after acute MI have evidence of systemic embolisation, and the incidence of stroke is between 1.5–3.5% of patients. The larger the infarct, the greater the chance of mural thrombosis (presumably due to the larger area of damaged endocardium, with platelet deposition thereon) and embolism. This is a particular risk if the thrombus is pedunculated rather than a laminar mural thrombus. A large pedunculated thrombus may still represent a considerable risk during anticoagulant therapy.

98 **i.** The ECG shows ventricular tachycardia (VT).
ii. Positive concordance in the chest leads and the R wave being higher than the R′ in V1 (higher 'left rabbit's ear') point to a left ventricular origin of the tachycardia.
iii. In the context of the question, the arrhythmia is probably still within the time frame of myocardial reperfusion. If the patient is symptomatic, DC electrical cardioversion is the quickest and most effective therapy. An intravenous bolus of lignocaine is also very likely to be effective, as is a bolus injection of magnesium sulphate.
iv. An episode of VT four weeks after myocardial infarction has a quite different prognosis. It occurs in about 5% of patients and is an independent risk factor for subsequent sudden cardiac death. There is a very good case for detailed investigation of this patient, with repeated Holter monitoring to assess the presence or frequency of ventricular premature beats or more complex ventricular arrhythmias and electrophysiological study to demonstrate inducible VT. The treatment options range from drug therapy, among which amiodarone is probably the most effective and least proarrhythmic, through catheter ablation, to implantation of an automatic cardioverter/defibrillator.

99 There is a double aortic knuckle, which is characteristic of coarctation of the aorta. The upper part is the dilated left subclavian artery and the lower part is the post-stenotic dilatation of the descending aorta. There is no evidence of rib notching on this chest radiograph, although it is characteristic of coarctation and is due to erosion of the under surface of ribs from dilated intercostal arteries. Rib notching is rare under the age of 10 years. The differential diagnosis of rib notching includes superior vena caval obstruction and neurofibromatosis. (See **91** and **150**.)

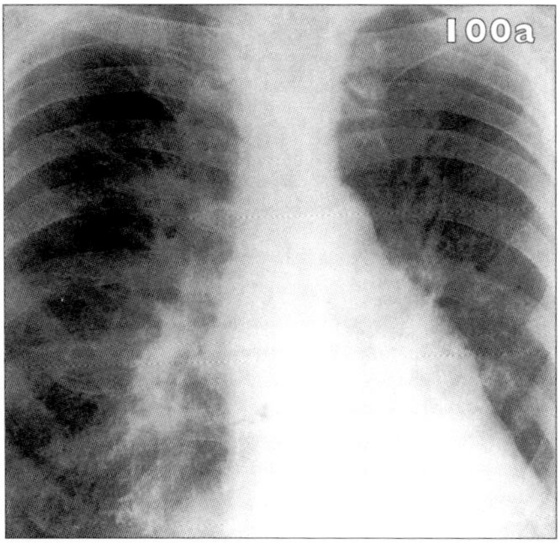

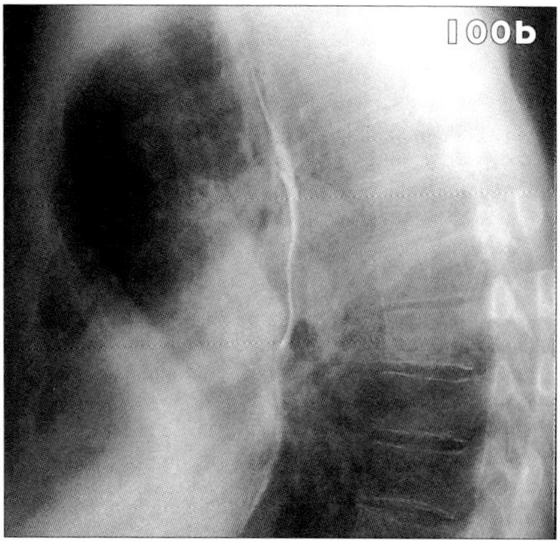

100 An asymptomatic 30-year-old man had a chest radiograph (**100a**) for insurance purposes. To his horror, when he read the printed report which accompanied the radiograph it described 'enlargement of the heart'. He urgently consulted a specialist, who requested another radiograph (**100b**). How did the specialist allay the young man's fears?

101 This 60-year-old patient had rheumatic fever as a child and has been followed in the cardiology clinic since.
i. What is the investigation?
ii. What two features of note can you see?
iii. What physical sign is likely to be related to the features you have noted?

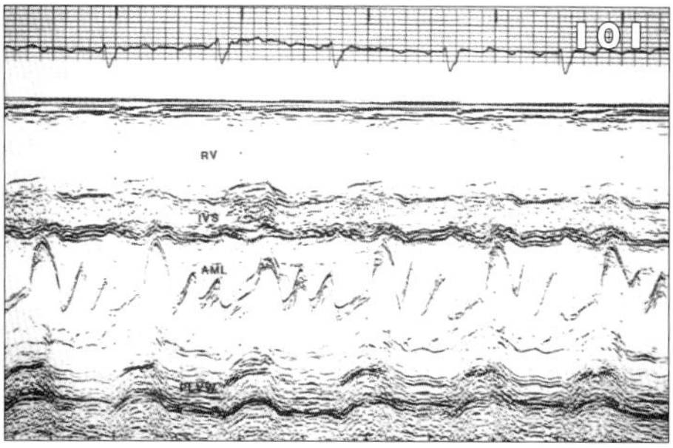

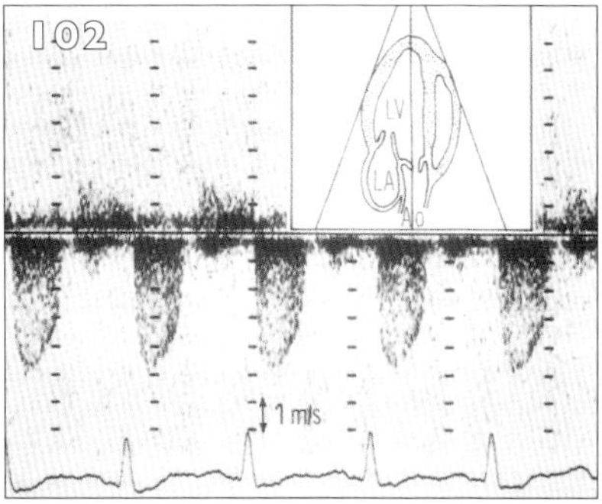

102 **i.** What is this investigation?
ii. What does it show?
iii. The peak velocity recorded was 4 m/s. What should you conclude?

100 Although the postero-anterior chest radiograph (**100a**) does show an increased cardiothoracic ratio, the lateral view (**100b**) shows that the sternum is depressed and the usual space between the chest wall and right atrium is reduced. The patient has pectus excavatum; the heart itself is entirely normal. Pectus excavatum can be recognised from the postero-anterior view alone. The heart is usually displaced to the left and the intervertebral discs can be seen equally clearly all the way down behind the heart, because of the narrow depth of the chest.

101 **i.** The investigation is an M mode echocardiogram.
ii. The patient has chronic aortic regurgitation. The features referred to are dilatation of the left ventricular chamber and diastolic fluttering of the anterior mitral valve leaflet. The latter is readily detectable by the M mode method; however, its presence and severity do not correlate with the degree of regurgitation. It is a useful sign in that, on imaging, the aortic valve sometimes appears normal despite being severely regurgitant. Doppler echocardiography is the optimal method for the non-invasive demonstration of aortic regurgitation, while 2D echo can often identify the cause. The enlargement of the left ventricular chamber indicates a gradual response to chronic volume loading of the ventricle.
iii. The physical sign corresponding to the mitral valve fluttering is the Austin Flint murmur (see **92**). This must be distinguished from any concomitant mitral valve stenosis; echocardiography can readily achieve this.

102 **i.** and **ii.** This is a continuous-wave Doppler study of a stenosed aortic valve. Although pulsed-wave Doppler is the mode of choice to locate the precise site of increase in flow velocity (i.e. at the level of the aortic valve, subvalvar or supravalvar), the high velocities of flow associated with even moderate degrees of valve stenosis cause problems of quantification due to aliasing. For this reason, to quantify flow velocity continuous-wave Doppler is used.
iii. From the measured velocity, the peak pressure gradient can be obtained using the modified Bernoulli equation, $\{P_1 - P_2 = 4[(V_2)^2 - (V_1)^2]\}$, where P_1 is the peak distal pressure, P_2 the peak proximal pressure, V_1 the pre-obstruction peak velocity, and V_1 the post-obstruction peak velocity. V_1 is less than one in most cases, other than those of appreciable valvar incompetence; therefore $P_1 - P_2 \sim 4V_2{}^2$. In this case, the peak velocity is 4 m/s, thus the peak pressure gradient will be about 64 mmHg. This indicates that the stenosis is of moderate severity.

103 The pressure tracing recorded during catheterisation of an asymptomatic young woman (a frame of whose angiogram is shown here) revealed a gradient of 5 mmHg between the left atrium and left ventricle.

i. What is the diagnosis?
ii. Comment on the left atrial size.
iii. What is the natural history of this condition left untreated?

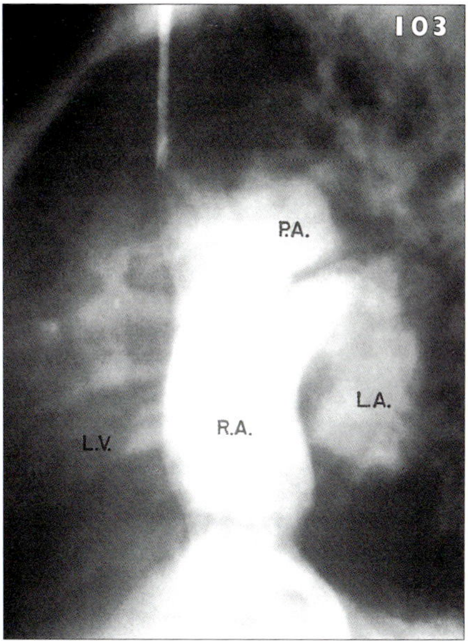

104 A 64-year-old patient, known to have undergone valve replacement 4 weeks previously, collapsed in the street and died before reaching hospital. A post-mortem was performed.

i. What does the illustration show?
ii. What other explanation might there have been if the operation had been carried out 15 years previously?

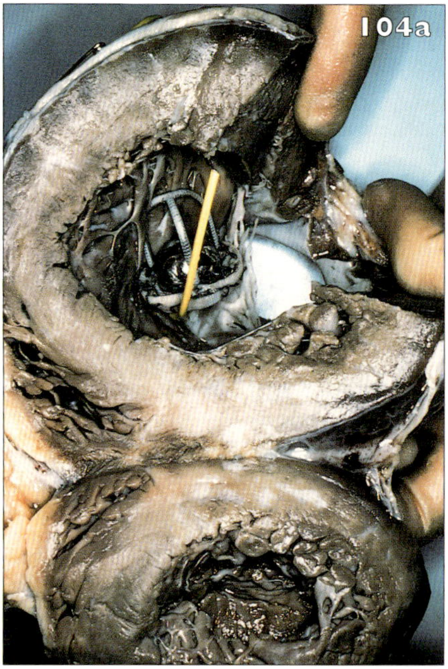

103 i. The presence of contrast in the left atrium, combined with the fact that a direct left atrial pressure is quoted in the question, show that (assuming the data did not result from a septal puncture) there is a communication between the right and left atria; i.e. there is an atrial septal defect (ASD). As well as this, there is a small, but significant, pressure gradient between the left atrium and left ventricle, i.e. mitral stenosis. The combination of ASD and acquired mitral stenosis constitutes Lutembacher's syndrome.
ii. The left atrium has been injected with contrast and can be seen to be dilated. Since the left atrium is vented through the ASD, the left atrial pressure is lower than in mitral stenosis without ASD, but the left-to-right shunt is increased and the left ventricular output reduced.
iii. Complications of the *untreated* condition reflect the underlying structural abnormalities. These are pulmonary vascular disease, systemic embolism and low cardiac output. Congestive heart failure is a probable ultimate development, occurring earlier if the mitral stenosis is severe.

104 i. Dehiscence of an aortic valve prosthesis is shown. The patient in question had a dehiscence of a prosthetic aortic valve (the natural valve was replaced with a Starr–Edwards prosthesis). The tissue at the site of attachment of the prosthetic valve ring was considered rather friable by the surgeon and, presumably as a consequence of this, adequate healing did not occur. If the patient had been seen before collapse, auscultation would probably have revealed a florid paravalvar leak. A similar case in which rocking of a loose valve prosthesis can clearly be seen is shown in these angio frames (**104b**).
ii. Strut fracture of the convex–concave model of the Bjork–Shiley tilting disc mechanical valves manufactured between 1976 and 1986 is still an occasional problem. Fracture of the outlet strut allows escape of the occluder, usually with a fatal outcome. Since the introduction of the monostrut, mechanical failure has become a very rare event.

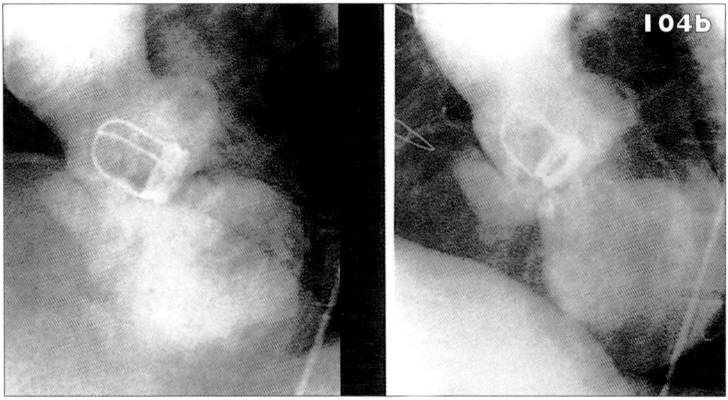
104b

105 **i.** What is this device?
ii. What are its indications and limitations?

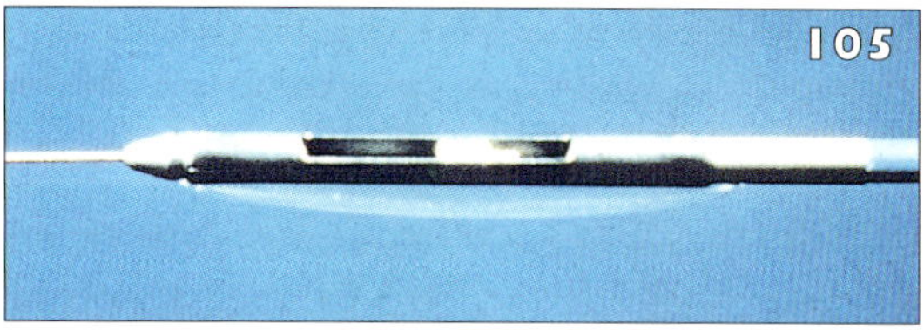

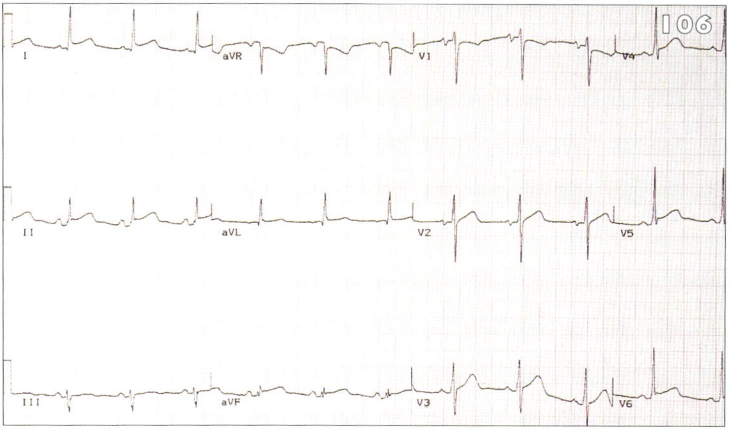

106 A 35-year-old man presents with a 6-hour history of central chest pain which, he has noticed, is worse on swallowing.
i. What is the diagnosis?
ii. What would be your next investigation

107 This 46-year-old patient had suffered from rheumatic fever. What is the abnormality on this M mode echocardiogram?

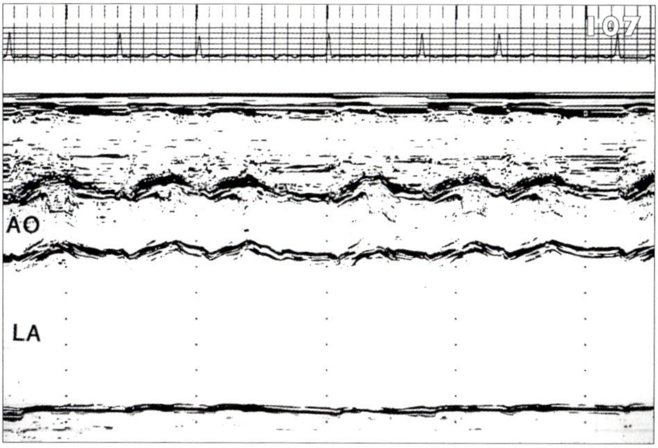

105 i. The device is an atherectomy catheter.
ii. Simpson's directional atherectomy catheter (a tube with a longitudinal opening along one side and a cutter sited within) was the first device to be employed in human coronary arteries. Its action is to shave the atheromatous material projecting into the vessel lumen and to collect the debris. It is indicated for larger arteries and eccentric proximal stenoses, especially those containing thrombus. Auth introduced a very high speed rotational device, the rotablator, which bores away at atheroma, releasing its (generally very fine) particles downstream. The indications for the use of this device are long eccentric lesions in small vessels, as well as for the recanalisation of totally occluded vessels. The transluminal extraction catheter of Stack is a flexible torque tube over a steerable wire which incorporates a conical cutter as well as a means of suction through the sides of the tip of the device. Laser devices have thus far had only limited success, but may be good for long, irregular and calcified lesions. However, the rate of restenosis for all these methods is equivalent to that for conventional percutaneous transluminal coronary angioplasty and the risks of the procedures may be higher.

106 i. The ECG shows ST segment elevation, concave-upwards in all the standard leads and the anterior chest leads. The diagnosis is acute pericarditis. In a classic case of acute pericarditis, chest pain is typically precordial, may be severe, and is usually associated with fever. The pain is worse on inspiration and exacerbated by coughing, swallowing, or any other movement.
ii. The most useful investigation is an echocardiogram. This permits any pericardial effusion to be detected, localised and quantified. Both left and right ventricular function can also be assessed. A chest radiograph would not necessarily be helpful in that, more likely than not, it will be normal, with enlargement of the heart shadow only being obvious in the presence of a pericardial effusion of >250 ml. Besides these, and in addition to baseline values of the full blood count and blood biochemistry, a wide range of other investigations could be suggested to help define the underlying cause of the pericarditis. These include acute and convalescent viral titres, Paul–Bunnell test, cold agglutinins for mycoplasma and Legionella, auto-antibodies (including antinuclear factor), levels of complement components and of immune complexes, thyroid function tests, Mantoux test, sputum microscopy, culture and sensitivity. Uncommonly, a diagnostic pericardial tap will be positive for tuberculosis. Microscopy, culture and sensitivity of the aspirate, as well as Ziehl–Neelsen staining of any cellular component for mycobacteria, are necessary, but usually the diagnosis has to be confirmed after culture. Most cases of acute pericarditis are idiopathic, of presumed but unproven viral origin.

107 This is an M mode echocardiogram through the aortic valve and left atrium. The obvious abnormality is a dilated atrium, which should not exceed 4 cm (four squares on the echocardiogram shown). The aortic valve is normal and assumes a box shape in systole. The dilated atrium suggests the possibility of underlying rheumatic mitral valve disease or left ventricular failure.

108 A 52-year-old retired army sergeant was referred to hospital for further investigation of back pain. The pain was felt chiefly between the shoulder blades and had become chronic (of at least 6 months' duration). The examining doctor felt proud of himself for deducing the patient's military origins from the firm, regular, stamp of the old soldier's step as he came into the consulting room. However, he found the radiograph (**108a**) harder to explain.

i. Can you help the doctor reach a diagnosis?

ii. What investigations would you do?

iii. What is the differential diagnosis?

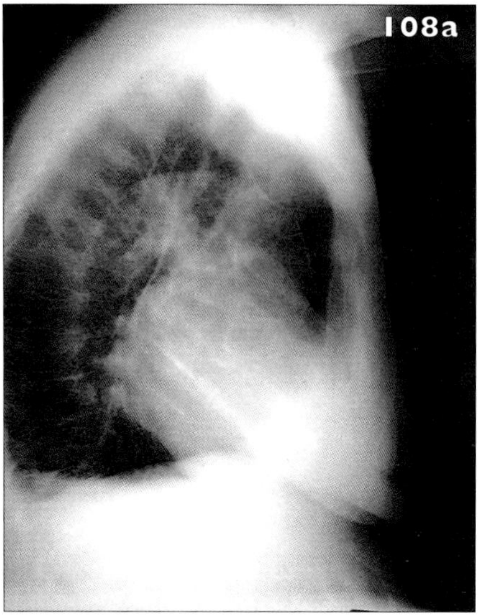

108a

109 This 22-year-old woman presented to the emergency department complaining of palpitations and breathlessness.

i. What is the ECG diagnosis?

ii. How might you treat this acute episode?

iii. How would you investigate this woman and what options are available to manage recurrent episodes?

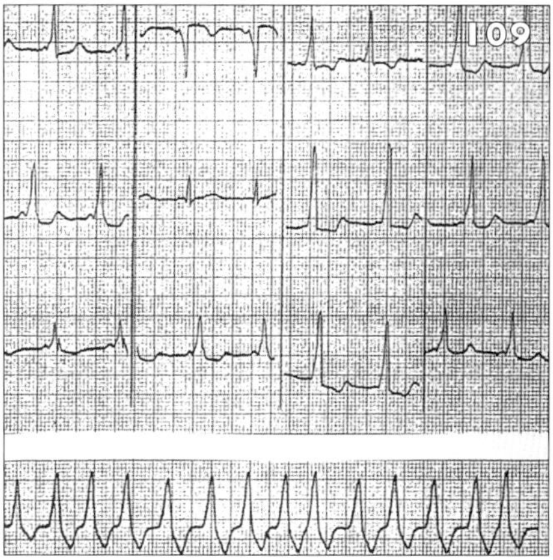

109

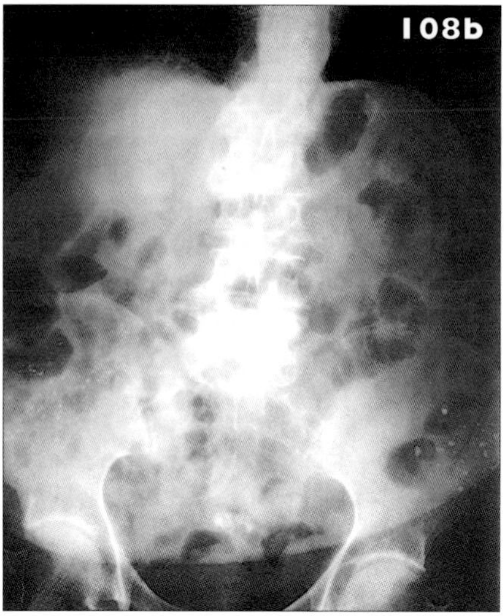

108 i. The lateral chest radiograph (**108a**) shows a calcified, dilated ascending aorta. The description of the pain is consistent with pressure upon the spine due to an aneurysm of the ascending aorta. The stamping gait probably owes more to tabes dorsalis acquired off-duty than to the persistence of parade ground skills. Thus, the underlying diagnosis is syphilitic aortitis. The ascending aorta is the classic site for syphilitic aortic aneurysms. Aortic regurgitation is very common in patients who present with syphilitic aortic aneurysms. Coronary ostial stenoses are also associated with both syphilitic aortic aneurysms and aortic regurgitation. A second radiograph (**108b**) shows signs of previous treatment for syphilis in the form of intramuscular bismuth injections.
ii. The diagnosis should be confirmed by Venereal Disease Research Laboratories (VDRL) and *Treponema pallidum* haemagglutination assay (TPHA) tests. The condition of the aorta would best be assessed by transoesophageal echocardiography.
iii. The differential diagnosis includes other causes of aortitis (e.g. Reiter's syndrome, cystic medial necrosis, and degenerative aneurysmal dilatation in association with atherosclerosis).

109 i. On the resting ECG, a ∂ wave and positive R wave can be seen in lead V1. The PR interval is also shorter than normal (<100 ms). Together these features point to a diagnosis of Wolff–Parkinson–White (WPW) syndrome. Since the ∂ wave is so clearly seen in leads V1–V3, the sub-diagnosis is WPW Type A, i.e. the accessory bundle is on the left side. The ECG during palpitation shows atrial fibrillation (AF) with broadened QRS complexes and a very fast ventricular response.
ii. In the emergency situation, with haemodynamic compromise, DC cardioversion is the treatment of choice. With a little more time available, intravenous amiodarone (e.g. 300 mg over 1 hour followed by 900 mg over the next 23 hours) is also very effective. It is extremely important to remember *not* to administer either digoxin or verapamil under these circumstances, as both can precipitate ventricular fibrillation.
iii. The development of AF in this woman merits catheter ablation or surgical resection of the accessory pathway after electrophysiological mapping, since it has already been shown that an excessively fast ventricular response to the atrial fibrillation can occur.

110 **i.** List three abnormalities on this ECG.
ii. The patient had rheumatic fever 20 years previously. What is the probable diagnosis?

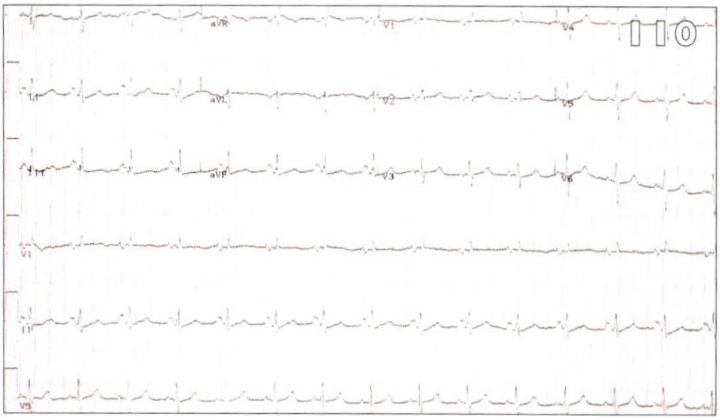

111 A 75-year-old woman complained of dizzy spells and had collapsed on two occasions.
i. What is the underlying diagnosis?
ii. What different treatment options are available?
iii. What is the incidence of this problem?

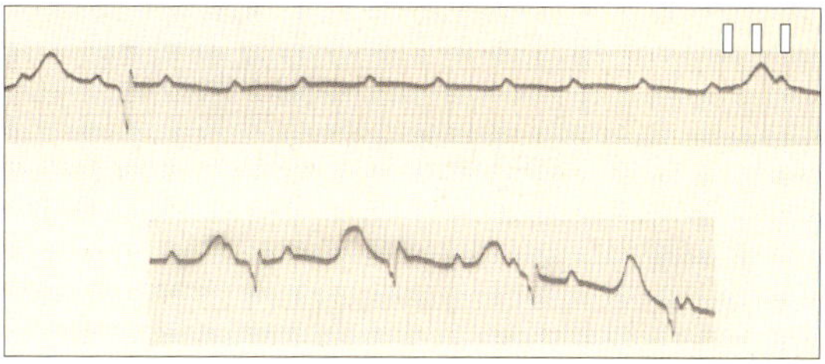

112 A 25-year-old asymptomatic woman was found to have an ejection sound and systolic murmur at and above the left sternal edge, as well as a widely split S2.
i. What is the likely cause of this woman's murmur?
ii. What procedure is being performed?

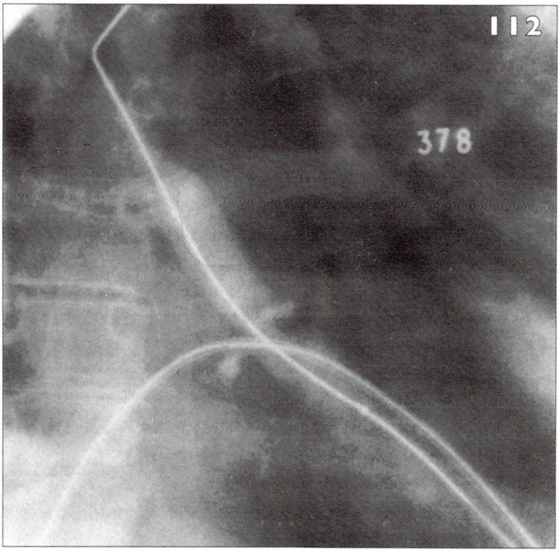

110 i. Three abnormalities are right axis deviation, P mitral is seen clearly in lead II and the P wave is biphasic in V1 (both these ECG findings are suggestive of left atrial enlargement), and there is a dominant R wave in V1 along with deep S waves in leads V5 and V6, which reflect right ventricular hypertrophy.
ii. The most probable diagnosis is rheumatic mitral valve disease, which would explain the left atrial enlargement. Pulmonary hypertension has caused a persistent high afterload on the right ventricle and resulted in hypertrophy. These ECG changes can also be produced in ostium secundum atrial septal defect and atrial myxoma.

111 i. The electrocardiogram shows a few normally conducted P waves, but these are followed by a run of several P waves with no ensuing QRS complex. This is usually due to fibrosis of the central bundle branches (Lenègre's disease) and the coronary arteries are often normal. Although no clinical details are given regarding the dizzy spells and two episodes of collapse, these often give clues to the underlying cause, with an absence of warning signs, short duration of unconsciousness (seconds) with rapid recovery, marked pallor during an attack, and a hot flush during recovery being characteristic.
ii. There is no medical therapy for Stokes–Adams attacks; a permanent pacing system is mandatory. If atrial function is not impaired, then a dual chamber system (DDD mode) enables a more physiological heart beat to be produced, although often a VVI system will be adequate. (*NB* Coronary angiography should be considered, especially in younger subjects, since myocardial ischaemia secondary to coronary artery disease may be the cause of the impaired intracardiac conduction.)
iii. The incidence of acquired complete heart block in those over 70 years of age is approximately 2/1000 of the population. It should not be 'left alone', as the prognosis untreated is very poor; for example, 35–50% mortality at 1 year after diagnosis, as compared to a 1-year mortality of <5% when paced.

112 i. The woman represents a typical case of pulmonary valve stenosis, which commonly occurs as an isolated lesion (7% of cases of congenital abnormalities of the heart) as well as in combination with more complex lesions (e.g. as in Fallot's tetralogy). Pulmonary stenosis is commonly asymptomatic, even with moderately severe right ventricular outflow obstruction, since right ventricular function usually remains good, the tricuspid valve competent and sinus rhythm preserved. On auscultation of such patients, a pulmonary ejection sound and systolic murmur can be heard and the pulmonary component of the second heart sound (P2) is delayed and soft. This permits an assessment of the pulmonary stenosis severity as mild (or no worse than mild-to-moderate). As the stenosis severity increases, A2 becomes obscured by the more prolonged systolic murmur. P2 is yet more delayed and becomes softer. In severe pulmonary stenosis, the ejection sound disappears and P2 is inaudible.
ii. A percutaneous pulmonary balloon valvoplasty is being performed in a more severe and younger patient. The results of this measure compare favourably with surgery, with a significant reduction in trans-pulmonic gradient being achieved, along with electrocardiographic evidence of regression of right ventricular hypertrophy.

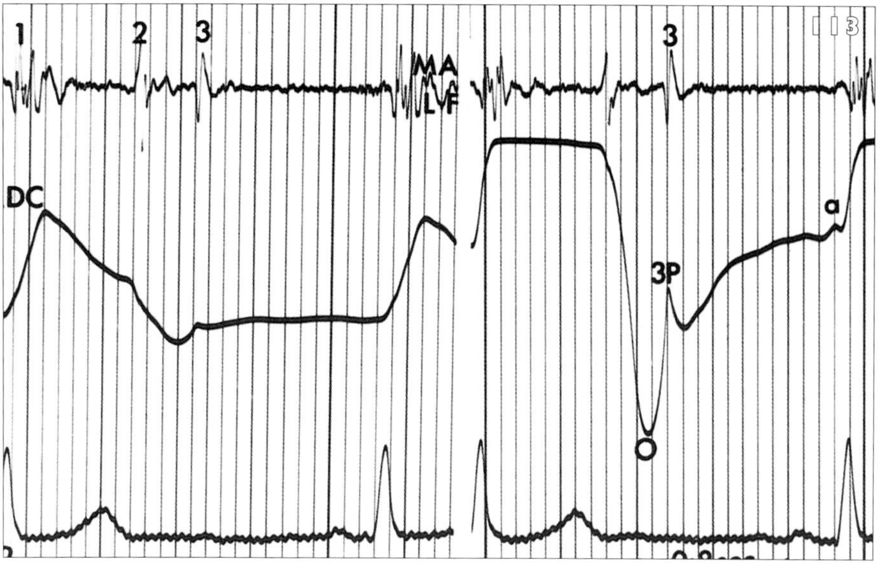

113 This finding was noted on auscultation of the chest of an asymptomatic healthy 24-year-old woman undergoing an insurance medical.
i. What is the finding?
ii. What produces it?

114 A 60-year-old patient presents with a 4-day history of high fever and breathlessness. On examination she is extremely unwell and peripherally cyanosed, with a temperature of 38.5°C and a sinus tachycardia. The apex beat is displaced and thrusting and there is a loud murmur of mitral regurgitation. On auscultation of the lungs there are fine inspiratory crackles throughout the lung fields. Urgent echocardiography demonstrates a large, floppy vegetation on the posterior mitral valve leaflet and severe mitral regurgitation with preserved systolic left ventricular function. Shortly afterwards she had a transient episode of dysphasia and left facial weakness.
i. Briefly list the management strategy in four steps.
ii. What are the indications for surgery in infective endocarditis?

113 i. The phonocardiogram (upper trace) shows a third heart sound.
ii. During the rapid filling phase of diastole, the ventricular chamber expands rapidly, but the expansion, especially in the long axis, is halted abruptly. This is the most widely accepted reason for the third heart sound. It can be seen from the apexcardiogram (lower trace) that the third sound coincides with the peak of the rapid filling wave. It occurs about 0.15 s after closure of the aortic valve. This time interval – longer than that between the second sound and an opening snap – helps to distinguish the third heart sound from the latter, as does the third sound's lower pitch. An audible third sound is also a feature of a normal heart in a high-output state, such as hyperthyroidism or pregnancy. It is also found in a number of pathological states associated with left ventricular dysfunction, such as dilated cardiomyopathy, whether ischaemic in aetiology or idiopathic. It also occurs in non-rheumatic mitral regurgitation. A *right* ventricular third heart sound is probably the basis of the 'pericardial' knock heard in constrictive pericarditis, which also involves the underlying myocardium.

114 i. The patient has severe haemodynamic compromise due to severe valvar regurgitation. She requires urgent mitral valve replacement, but prior to surgery she needs the following:
(a) 100% oxygen, provided she does not have severe chronic airways disease.
(b) Intravenous diuretics to relieve the pulmonary oedema. If the blood pressure is low inotropes are indicated; there may also be a place for intravenous nitrates to reduce afterload on the left ventricle and further ameliorate the pulmonary oedema.
(c) Haemodynamic support with vasodilator agents to improve forward cardiac output.
(d) After several blood cultures have been taken, she should be commenced on intravenous antibiotics. This is a very acute presentation and therefore it is necessary to cover both staphylococcal and streptococcal infection. High-dose penicillin and flucloxacillin should be commenced as soon as possible. It is also advisable to couple this with an aminoglycoside, usually gentamicin.

ii. Indications for surgery are as follows:
(a) Severe valvar regurgitation causing haemodynamic compromise.
(b) Large vegetations, particularly if there has already been clinical evidence of embolism.
(c) Failure to respond to antibiotics. This is manifested in persistent fever, continuing clinical deterioration and persistently raised C-reactive protein. The most common cause for this is a resistant organism or localised paravalvar abscess formation.
(d) Conduction abnormalities suggest a septal abscess, which in particular can complicate aortic valve endocarditis.
(e) Prosthetic valve endocarditis is difficult to treat medically if the infection presents early after surgery, because the infecting organisms are usually resistant to the usual antibiotics. Late prosthetic valve endocarditis is caused by sensitive organisms.

115 A 68-year-old man was brought to the family doctor by his wife. She said that he had become considerably less energetic over the previous year, moved slowly and was rather tremulous. An ECG was recorded and is shown. Comment upon the ECG appearances.

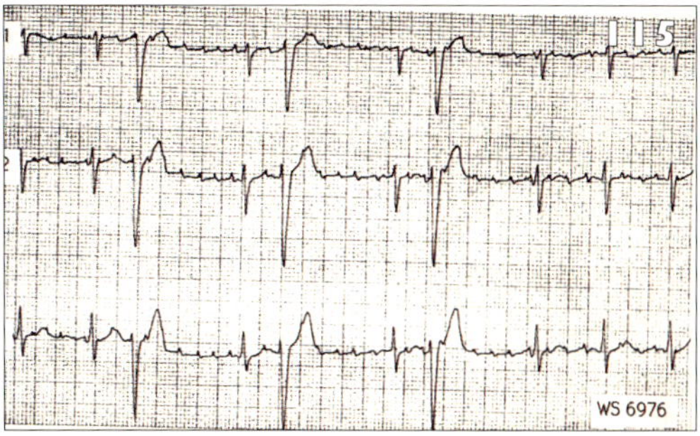

116 A 60-year-old man with a 3-day history of severe and rapidly worsening breathlessness was admitted as an emergency, underwent echocardography and was taken to the cardiac catheterisation laboratory the same day. The pressures measured are shown on the right.

Chamber	*Pressure (mmHg)*
Pulmonary capillary wedge (mean)	30
Pulmonary artery	40/20
Right ventricle	42/8
Right atrium	a, 7; v, 6
Left ventricle	180/30
Aorta	120/70

i. What is the diagnosis?
ii. What event has probably triggered the crisis?
iii. What are the relative merits of medical and surgical treatments under these circumstances?

117 **i.** What is the rationale for intra-aortic balloon counterpulsation?
ii. What benefits can it provide?
iii. When should it not be used?

118 What does this ECG rhythm strip demonstrate?

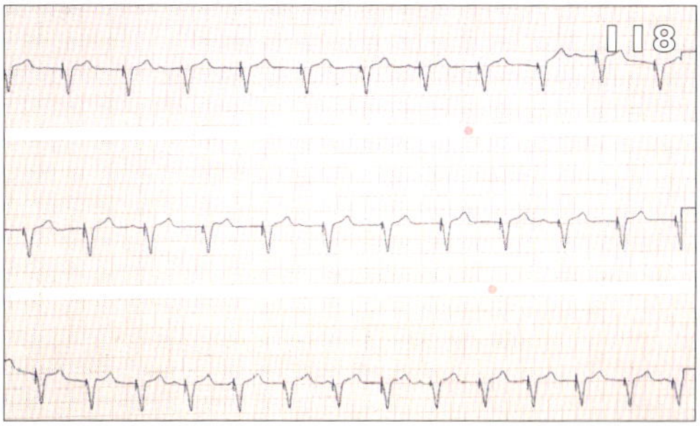

115 The small deflections on the ECG are not P waves in a case of complete heart block, but deflections due to the Parkinsonian tremor. The rest of the ECG is normal.

116 i. In practice, the diagnosis was clinched by the initial echocardiogram; the cardiac catheterisation was performed to define the coronary anatomy; however, the opportunity was also taken to acquire the cardiac pressures shown. Considering the data, the pulmonary capillary wedge pressure is raised to 30 mmHg, but the pulmonary artery pressure and right ventricular pressure are only mildly raised at 40/20 mmHg and 42/8 mmHg respectively. The right atrial pressure is very slightly raised, with an a of 7 mmHg and v of 6 mmHg (for normal ranges, see *Appendix*). This patient had aortic stenosis (there is a gradient of 60 mmHg across the aortic valve) and had developed mitral regurgitation acutely – hence the raised left ventricular end-diastolic pressure, which is equal to the pulmonary wedge.
ii. The acute development of mitral regurgitation in this case is statistically most probably due to degenerative mitral valve prolapse. The high left ventricular pressure caused by the pre-existing aortic stenosis may have promoted chordal rupture.
iii. Medical management has nothing to offer in this rare emergency. Vasodilators are often tried, because of the evidence of heart failure, but could have disastrous effects. Urgent surgical correction of both valves (e.g. mitral valve repair and aortic valve replacement) is life-saving, but first the reason for the sudden deterioration needs to be suspected and the diagnosis rapidly made or confirmed by echocardiography.

117 i. In intra-aortic balloon counterpulsation, inflation of the balloon is synchronised with left ventricular activity by means of the ECG. It inflates in diastole, thereby increasing diastolic blood pressure and improving coronary artery perfusion pressure. The deflation during systole unloads a failing ventricle by sudden production of a low impedance sink. Overall, cardiac output can be increased by up to one-third.
ii. This technique can make all the difference, for example, in patients with cardiogenic shock or in helping the patient through a definitive procedure, such as percutaneous transluminal coronary angioplasty or coronary bypass grafting.
iii. Contraindications to the use of aortic balloon counterpulsation include significant renal and hepatic failure, peripheral vascular disease, cerebrovascular disease, coagulopathy, severe infection and disseminated cancer.

118 This is a paced ventricular rhythm (QRS complexes are preceded by a pacing spike). All the pacing spikes are followed by a QRS complex, suggesting that there is no evidence of failure to capture. Single chamber ventricular stimulation was the pacing mode established as a life-saving measure in the early 1960s, but this type of system cannot maintain atrial transport and is associated with haemodynamic disturbance in over 10% of patients. Congestive cardiac failure occurs more often if single chamber ventricular pacing is begun in patients with bradyarrhythmias in whom the atria contract effectively prior to pacemaker implantation. Single chamber ventricular pacing is recommended in patients with bradyarrhythmias who are in atrial fibrillation, because here atrial contraction does not contribute to cardiac output.

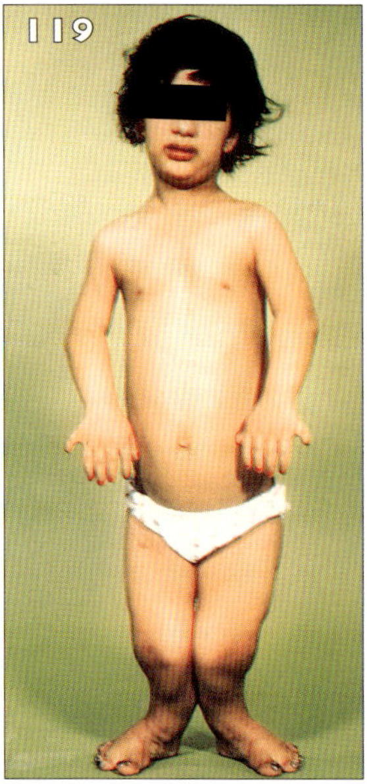

119 This child has a heart murmur.
i. What is the disorder?
ii. What is the mode of inheritance?
iii. Give a likely cause for the murmur.

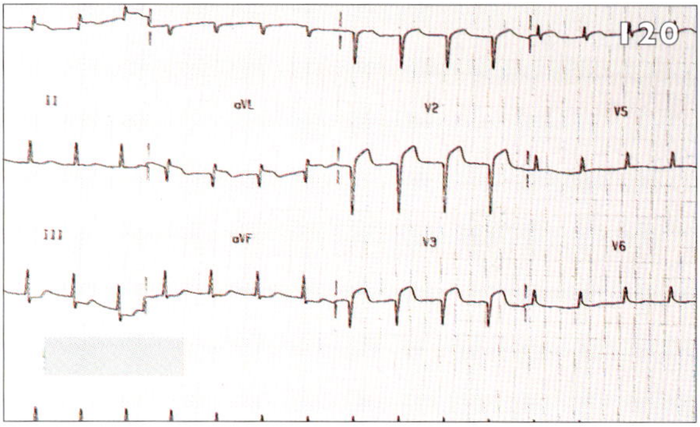

120 A 60-year-old man, whose only previous medical condition of note had been maturity-onset diabetes, collapsed at a bus stop. He was breathless and sweaty but experienced no pain.
i. What has happened to the patient?
ii. How common is this clinical scenario?

121 A 36-year-old man underwent repeat cardiac catheterisation because of persistent, somewhat atypical chest pain, 4 years after three-vessel coronary artery bypass grafting.
i. What is shown?
ii. Are you surprised at the condition of this structure 4 years after the original operation?
iii. One of the vein grafts was blocked. What do you think about an operation to regraft?

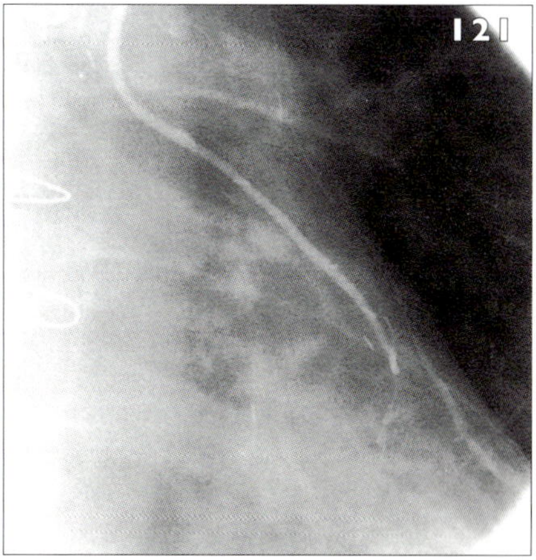

119 i. This child has Ellis–van Creveld syndrome.
ii. It is recessively inherited.
iii. Ellis–van Creveld syndrome (also known as chondroectodermal dysplasia) is a rare chondrodysplastic disorder, most common among the Amish. The disorder is characterised by short-limbed dwarfism due to metaphyseal dysplasia with polydactyly and dysplasia of the nails and teeth. Of these cases, 50% have associated cardiac malformations, usually endocardial cushion defects ranging from mild to a single (common) atrium and partial atrioventricular canal. About 20% of cases have associated coarctation, hypoplastic left heart, or patent ductus arteriosus. At the biochemical level, a defect in the extracellular matrix has been hypothesised. Prenatal diagnosis can be aided by the detection of polydactyly by ultrasound.

120 i. The ST segment elevation in the anterior chest leads and developing Q waves show that the man has had an acute anterior myocardial infarction.
ii. The incidence of painless ('silent') myocardial infarction is probably at least 25% of patients under 70 years of age who experience myocardial infarction. The incidence is considerably higher in older patients and especially in diabetics. The fact that the infarct and the associated myocardial ischaemia are silent is a poor prognostic indicator. Although, in general, the basis of the silence of silent myocardial ischaemia is far from agreed, it seems probable that autonomic neuropathy has an aetiological role in the silent ischaemia of diabetic patients. Angiography in a patient such as this might be expected to reveal severe coronary artery disease, with an anterior descending artery occlusion.

121 i. Shown is an angiogram of a left internal mammary artery (LIMA) graft to the left anterior descending (LAD) coronary artery. The metal clips on the side branches of the mobilised artery are characteristic. The graft is patent, filling the distal LAD territory.
ii. Statistically, it is more likely than not that a LIMA graft would be patent 4 years after the bypass operation. Arterial grafts have a better rate of survival, especially at more than 10 years after surgery.
iii. The patent internal mammary artery graft confers a relatively good prognosis. The risk of disrupting this graft during a repeat sternotomy makes reoperation inadvisable on account of a single blocked vein graft, so medical management should be pursued. However, further investigation to assess the functional significance of the occlusion of the vein graft is advisable. Thus, stress echo could demonstrate whether a regional wall motion abnormality was present in the territory of the blocked vein graft. Risk factor management should also receive close attention, e.g. cessation of smoking and lowering of cholesterol levels.

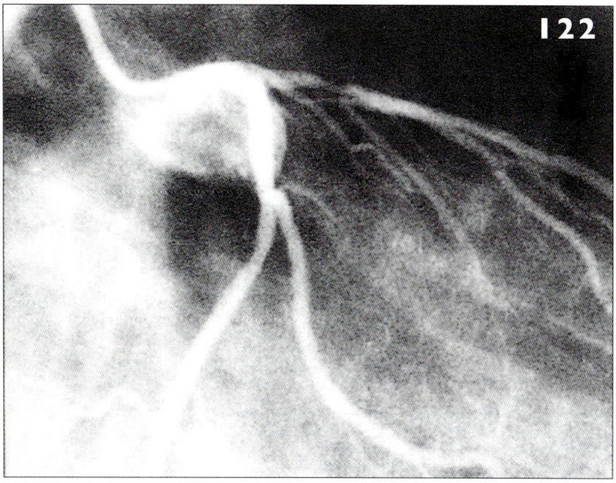

122 A 26-year-old rock singer was brought into the emergency department complaining of severe central chest pain, which commenced in the small hours of the morning after a post-concert party. In the course of investigation by the cardiologists, this angiogram was obtained. Suggest an explanation for the events described.

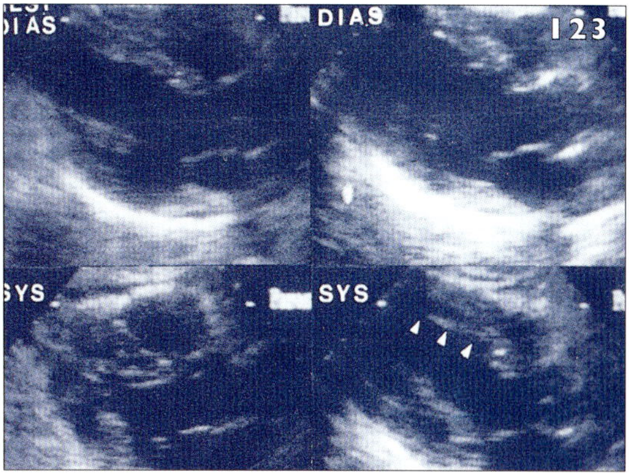

123 A patient with left bundle branch block (LBBB) on the resting ECG underwent a procedure involving intravenous infusion of adenosine with simultaneous echocardiography. The images at rest and at the peak tolerable infusion are shown.
i. What are the indications for this method of investigation?
ii. What is the mechanism of action of the pharmacological stressor in this case?
iii. What clinical information can you derive in this specific case?

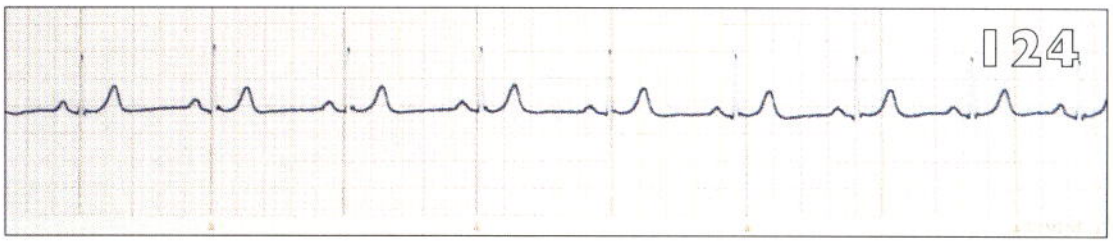

124 A 60-year-old man collapsed at a bus stop outside his local hospital. A passer-by attempted basic resuscitation and an emergency team was soon on hand. On examination, there were no palpable arterial pulses, audible heart sounds, or respiratory efforts. The trace shown was obtained via the paddles of the defibrillator.
i. Identify the rhythm.
ii. Explain the mechanisms and give five possible causes.

122 The angiogram shows a tight focal stenosis (>95% of luminal diameter) of the proximal left anterior descending (LAD) coronary artery. The rest of the left coronary system appears to be smooth and free of disease. The sequence of events in this case would be as follows. The rock singer used cocaine, which he 'snorted'. In addition to its stimulatory effects on the central nervous system, producing euphoria and, at times, hallucinations, cocaine has a number of cardiovascular effects. It can provoke ventricular arrhythmias and is also a powerful vasoconstrictor. The latter effect can cause coronary artery spasm, which can, in turn, lead to acute myocardial infarction, as in this patient. At the arterial level, the stenosis shown probably results from focal coronary spasm causing local damage to the arterial intima. Platelet deposition and thrombosis upon the site of injury develop the lesion and the process is furthered by impaired endothelial function and reduced nitric oxide synthesis.

123 **i.** A pharmacological stress echocardiogram has been performed, in this case with adenosine. Stress echocardiograms are being employed increasingly for the diagnosis of coronary artery disease; the method is more specific than an exercise ECG and, if an inotrope such as dobutamine is used, it also allows assessment of global and regional myocardial contractile reserve. Predictably, it is of considerable value in cases in which there are difficulties of ECG interpretation, such as LBBB. The use of scoring systems, based upon whether the separate myocardial segments become hypokinetic, akinetic, or dyskinetic, permits (at least) semi-quantitative comparison between subjects.
ii. Adenosine is a powerful vasodilator which acts, via specific A_2 purinergic receptors, upon the coronary microcirculation, especially below the level of vessels 500 μm in diameter. The reduction of resistance downstream evokes a large increase in blood flow through the myocardium, except in segments supplied by stenosed epicardial arteries.
iii. The illustration shows a reduction in the contraction in the anterior free wall of the left ventricle.

124 **i.** Despite the complete absence of cardiac output, the ECG complexes are normal; this is 'electromechanical dissociation' (pulseless electrical activity), i.e. the normal electrical activity is dissociated from the appropriate mechanical pumping action of the heart.
ii. The mechanisms of electromechanical dissociation are leakage of blood out of the circulation (e.g. due to internal haemorrhage, ventricular rupture, or aortic dissection), 'short circuiting' of the circulation (e.g. rupture of the ventricular septum), pump failure (e.g. due to inability of the heart to contract effectively in cardiogenic shock due to myocardial infarction), inability of the heart to fill sufficiently in cardiac tamponade and tension pneumothorax, inadequate cardiac output due to reduced systemic blood pressure in hypothermia, and major obstruction to forward flow out of the heart (e.g. after massive pulmonary embolism).

125 A 30-year-old woman was admitted to hospital following an inferior myocardial infarction. She did not have a family history of ischaemic heart disease or any acquired risk factors. On examination she was unwell and had a high temperature, her heart rate was 110 b.p.m. and regular, and her blood pressure was 170/95 mmHg. She had several splinter haemorrhages on her finger nails. Auscultation of the heart revealed a soft pericardial rub, but the heart sounds were normal and there were no murmurs. Peripheral pulses were palpable and there was no evidence of peripheral oedema. Roth spots were present on examination of both fundi. On further enquiry the patient gave a history of night sweats and generalised myalgia for the previous 6 weeks. She had lost almost 10 kg in weight during this period. Investigations are shown at top, right.

Investigations

Full blood count:	
Hb	9 g/dl
WCC	15 x 10^9/l
Platelets	500 x 10^9/l
Serum creatinine	200 μmol/l (2.26 mg/dl)
C-reactive protein	100 mg/l

Chest radiograph normal

i. Suggest two possible diagnoses.
ii. List four tests which could help differentiate between your diagnoses.

126 A 55-year-old welder complained of worsening breathlessness over the course of about 4 months. On a particularly bad day he presented to the emergency department acutely short of breath. On auscultation, his heart sounds were normal, but basal crackles could be heard in the chest. The chest radiograph is shown; however, a subsequent stress ECG and echocardiogram were both normal. What is the diagnosis?

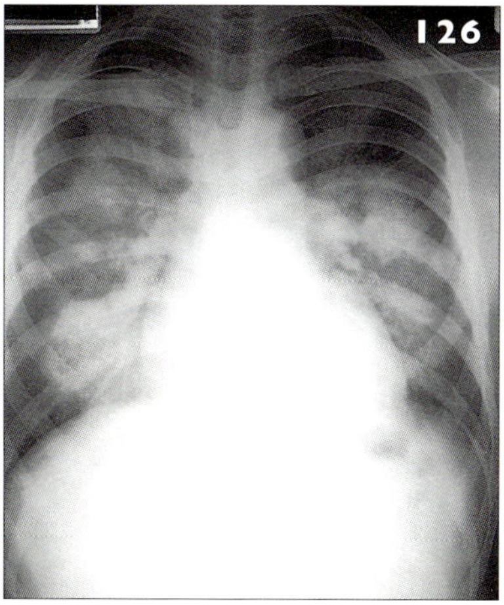

127 A 62-year-old man had an uncomplicated myocardial infarction 3 months ago, after which he had remained very well. Fasting serum lipids in clinic revealed a serum cholesterol of 8.2 mmol/l (317 mg/dl). Which two management steps would you take?

125 **i.** Two possible diagnoses are infective endocarditis and polyarteritis nodosa. **ii.** Blood cultures, echocardiography, serum antineutrophil cytoplasmic antibodies (ANCA), renal biopsy and coronary angiography may help define the diagnosis. Blood cultures and echocardiography help to establish a diagnosis of infective endocarditis. Serum ANCA may be positive in polyarteritis nodosa. Renal biopsy with immunofluorescent stains could differentiate glomerulonephritis due to polyarteritis nodosa from that due to the immune complexes of endocarditis. A coronary angiogram may demonstrate microaneurysms in polyarteritis nodosa.

The most probable diagnosis in a young woman presenting with this type of illness would be infective endocarditis complicated by a vegetation embolising into a coronary artery. Against this is the absence of a cardiac murmur, which is almost invariably present. She certainly has the systemic and vasculitic features of the disease and exhibits a possible embolic phenomenon. A generalised vasculitis could explain all the features in her history and examination. Note that Roth spots are a vasculitic phenomenon probably due to immune-complex deposition, and are not specific for endocarditis – they can occur in any type of vasculitis. The main feature which would deter the clinician from the diagnosis of polyarteritis nodosa is the woman's age and sex. Polyarteritis usually occurs in middle-aged males. The diagnosis is made by biopsies of the affected organs or by demonstrating microaneurysms in the renal, hepatic, intestinal, or coronary vessels.

126 The chest radiograph shows a normal cardiac silhouette. The lung fields have only some of the appearances of pulmonary oedema (e.g. fluffy shadowing peripherally, more so at the bases than at the apex), but there are no Kerley B lines and no upper lobe venous engorgement. The man has non-cardiogenic pulmonary oedema, due to inhalation of iron oxide during welding. In contrast to coal worker's pneumoconiosis and silicosis, in which there is progressive fibrosis of the lung parenchyma, iron oxide particles are inert and removal of the cause will lead to reversion to normality, since the particles are removed from the lungs by the mucociliary elevator or after transportation to the intrapulmonary and hilar lymph nodes.

127 The patient has unacceptable hypercholesterolaemia, which has long been known to be involved in the atherosclerotic process and is a major risk factor for coronary artery disease. In 1994 the 4S Simvastatin study clearly demonstrated that effective reduction of serum cholesterol with statin treatment reduced the risk of death and serious adverse events in approximately one-third of patients with ischaemic heart disease. The aim is to keep the serum cholesterol level below 5.2 mmol/l (200 mg/dl). This patient requires dietary advice with respect to pursuing a low lipid diet. This would probably reduce his serum cholesterol by about 10% and so still leave him with a very high serum cholesterol. Secondary causes of hypercholesterolaemia, such as diabetes mellitus, hypothyroidism, primary biliary cirrhosis, and alcohol excess, need to be checked and where possible treatment should be instigated. In this case, drug therapy proved necessary; the most effective drugs for hypercholesterolaemia are HMGCoA-reductase inhibitors or the statins.

128 This 20-year-old woman has been monitored by the cardiac clinic for 8 years. She hurried up two flights of stairs to get to her consultation and looked as shown. On examination, a fixed split second heart sound was the only abnormality found.

i. What is the diagnosis?

ii. What would you advise regarding the safety of her becoming pregnant?

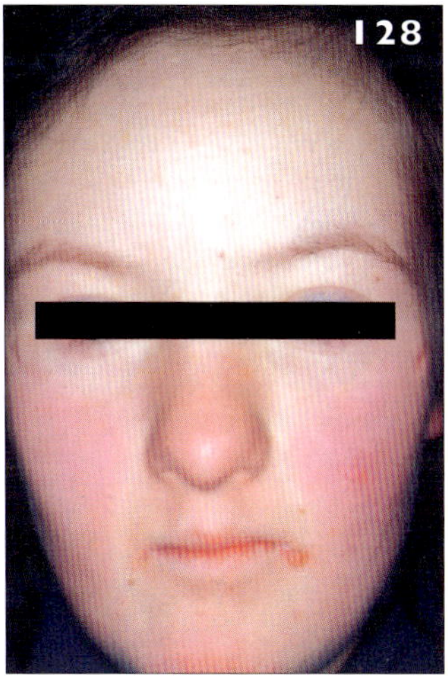

129 **i.** State three abnormalities in this chest radiograph.

ii. What is the probable diagnosis?

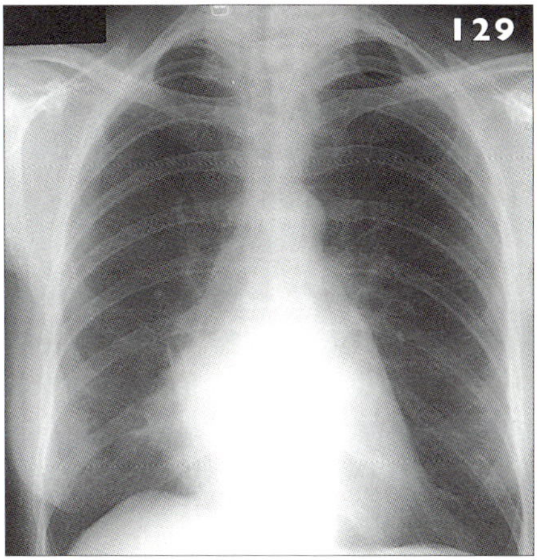

130 A 62-year-old man developed sudden onset of breathlessness and hypotension 48 hours after a myocardial infarction. On examination he was cold and clammy and the jugular venous pressure (JVP) was not raised. On auscultation of the heart there was a loud pan-systolic murmur at the apex.

i. Give two differential diagnoses.

ii. List two tests which would distinguish between your diagnoses.

128 i. The woman is clearly cyanosed. Enough clinical information is given to deduce that she has an atrial septal defect and shunt reversal on exertion, i.e. pulmonary hypertension.
ii. Pulmonary hypertension (e.g. as in Eisenmenger's syndrome) carries a high maternal mortality, with a range of 30–70%, the highest risk being in the early puerperium. Although fluid loading, inotropes and pressor agents have (at least some) clinical appeal, the outcome is often fatal. In contrast, cyanotic congenital heart disease in the absence of pulmonary hypertension is a low-risk lesion from the point of view of the mother, although prematurity of the newborn infant is common and there is an increased risk of fetal death. Pregnancy is therefore contraindicated in this case.

129 i. Three abnormalities are the left heart border is straightened, there is a double atrial shadow, and there is splaying of the carina – all features of an enlarged left atrium. Both main pulmonary arteries are prominent.
ii. The findings are consistent with a diagnosis of mitral stenosis, in which the earliest sign is left atrial enlargement. As the mitral stenosis progresses, dilatation of the upper pulmonary veins becomes obvious. The overall cardiac size increases on the radiograph as the right atrium dilates. Haemoptyses are due to recurrent rupture of small bronchial venules because of the very high back pressures. Small deposits of haemosiderin are seen as small white nodules mainly at the bases of the lungs, and are caused by leakage of blood into the lung parenchyma from pulmonary capillaries and venules.

130 i. Two differential diagnoses are acute mitral regurgitation (due to papillary muscle rupture) and acute ventricular septal defect.
ii. Echocardiography with colour flow and Doppler studies are diagnostic. The septal defect and the non-contracting, ruptured papillary muscle head can be visualised by echocardiography; colour flow studies solve the differential diagnosis. The severity of mitral regurgitation is difficult to quantify and clinical acumen is the best guide.

Swan-Ganz catheterisation with pressure and oxygen saturation measurements of the right heart and pulmonary artery is very useful in diagnosing acute ventricular septal defect. In this situation there is an increase in right heart pressures and a step up in oxygen saturation at the level of the right ventricle. Both mitral regurgitation and ventricular septal defect are recognised complications of myocardial infarction. Mitral regurgitation is a consequence of papillary muscle ischaemia or rupture and occurs following an inferior or posterior infarction. The patient develops rapid hypotension and pulmonary oedema. JVP is not commonly elevated and, on examination, there is usually a loud pan-systolic murmur and an accompanying systolic thrill. The murmur may be soft when the systolic gradient between the left ventricle and the left atrium becomes small. Ventricular septal defect complicates either anterior or inferior infarction and also presents in a similar manner. JVP is elevated due to acute pressure overload on the right ventricle and there is a pan-systolic murmur and an associated right ventricular heave. Early surgery is recommended in both situations.

131 A cardiologist was asked to see, as a matter of urgency, a patient who presented to his family doctor complaining of breathlessness. The ECG revealed signs of a recent anterior infarct, but the patient did not seem to know very much about this. In the course of a careful physical examination, the cardiologist observed the physical signs shown. What is the underlying diagnosis and what has happened?

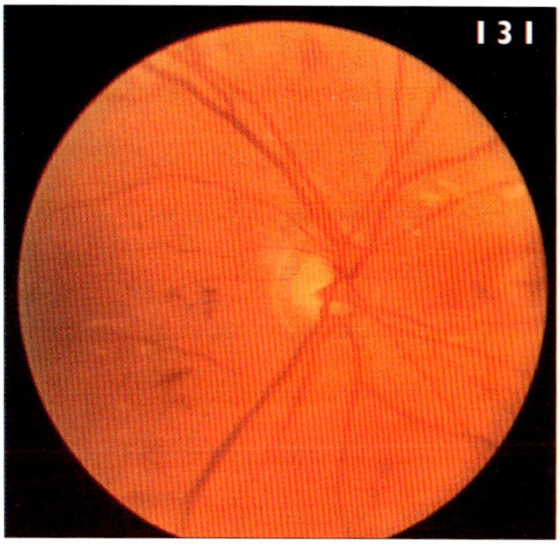

132 A 72-year-old man had undergone single vessel coronary artery bypass grafting surgery 8 years previously for worsening angina (he had not suffered myocardial infarction). Over the previous 4 months the chest pain had recurred and further investigations were instituted.

i. What investigation is shown?
ii. What anatomical information can you conclude from it?
iii. What is the natural history after this surgery?

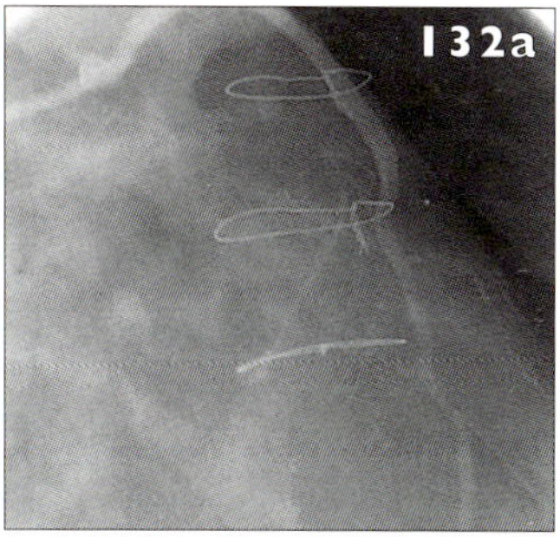

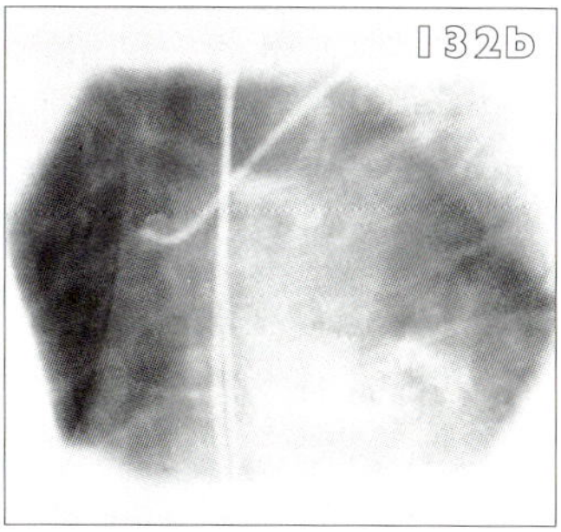

133 This tracing was obtained from a 65-year-old man who was reviewed routinely for medical.insurance He was not aware that he had anything the matter with him.

i. What abnormalities can you see on the ECG?
ii. Does anything need to be done?

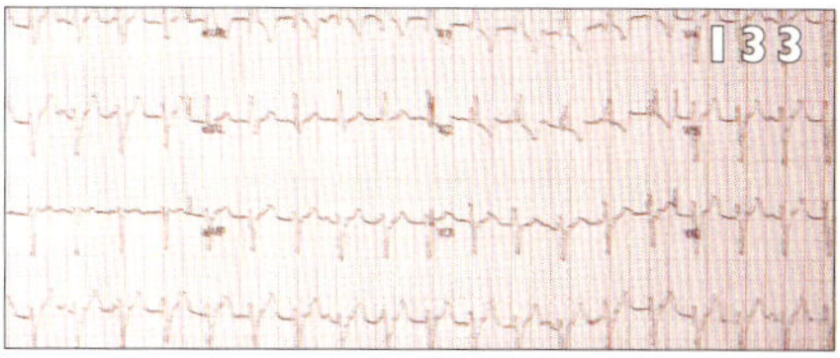

131 This fundoscopic image shows flame-shaped haemorrhages (superficial in the nerve layer), a few 'dot and blot' haemorrhages (deeper and between glial cells) and, especially in the inferior nasal quadrant and near the macula, a number of hard exudates (leakage around microvascular abnormalities). This is background diabetic retinopathy. The underlying diagnosis is diabetes mellitus. This patient had, indeed, sustained an anterior myocardial infarction, although it had been painless and the only symptom noted was an increase in breathlessness on exertion. Diabetic patients have a markedly increased rate of 'silent' (i.e. painless) myocardial infarction, the latter accounting for approximately 20% of infarcts in diabetic patients. The mechanism for the painlessness of this group of myocardial infarctions has been presumed to be autonomic neuropathy affecting the cardiac sympathetic afferent nerves (see **205**).

132 **i.** In the angiographic frame (**132a**), the left anterior descending artery (LAD) has been injected with contrast. In additon, a vein graft has been identified (**132b**).
ii. The native LAD is still patent, despite there being diffuse arterial disease distally. Injection into the stump of the vein graft shows it to be blocked.
iii. In general, 5-year and 10-year survival rates for patients after coronary artery bypass grafting are of the order of 90% and 50–75%, respectively [data from the Coronary Artery Surgery Study (CASS)]. Patients with internal mammary grafts do significantly better, with a lower rate of reinfarction, hospitalisation, and re-operation (two mammary artery grafts – left and right – appear to do even better). In the case of this patient, late occlusion of the vein graft is the most likely cause of the recent onset angina.

133 **i.** The mean frontal axis is abnormally leftwards (more than –30°). Thus, since there is no evidence of inferior infarction, the first diagnosis is left anterior hemiblock. In addition, rSR complexes are evident in leads V1 and V2 (the leads most oriented towards the right ventricle). The overall QRS complex duration is prolonged and so the first diagnosis is right bundle branch block. The reason for this M-shaped complex is that only after (a) depolarisation of the septum (from left to right, producing the initial r wave in V1) and (b) depolarisation of the left ventricular free wall (from right to left, producing the S wave in V1) does right ventricular depolarisation occur. When it does, it is due to the anomalous spread of depolarisation through the right ventricular free wall. This delayed left-to-right depolarisation produces the R′ wave (see **199**). In summary, the ECG shows right bundle branch block and left anterior hemiblock.
ii. Although both of these electrocardiographic features indicate dysfunction of the intracardiac pathways of conduction, since the man is asymptomatic, the current clinical view would be that there is no indication for pacing.

134 A 45-year-old man of previous good health was about to be discharged after orthopaedic treatment, having been admitted as an emergency after a road traffic accident His sternum had been fractured and was apparently healing well and a fracture of the right ulna had been reduced successfully. The orthopaedic intern noticed an extra physical sign. What did the intern find and how might it have come about?

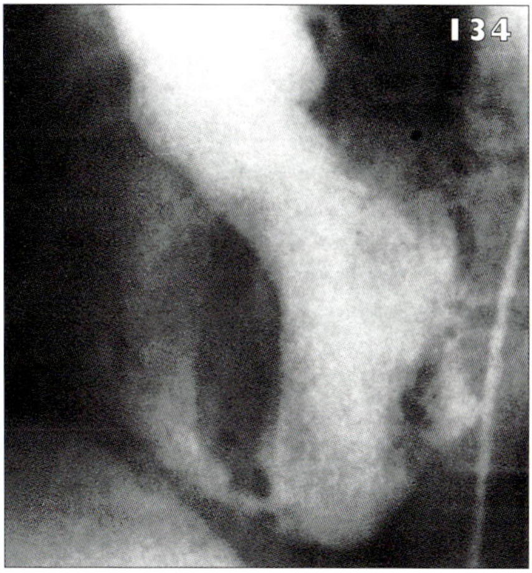

135 This is an ECG of a 45-year-old man taken during a routine insurance examination. He was asymptomatic and not on any medication. What are the abnormalities?

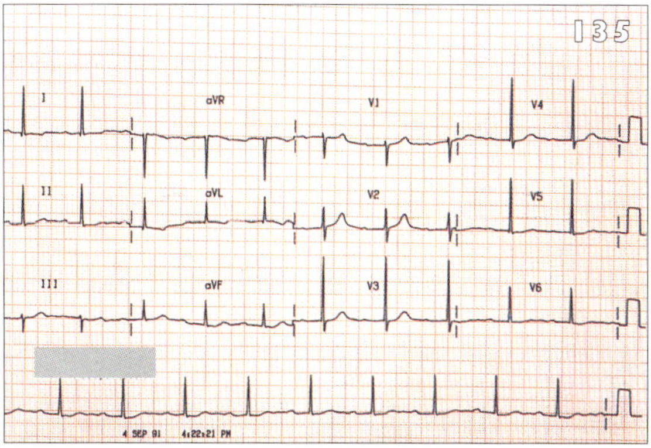

136 A 55-year-old man complained of breathlessness on exertion, but no chest pain.
i. What is the diagnosis?
ii. What is the treatment?

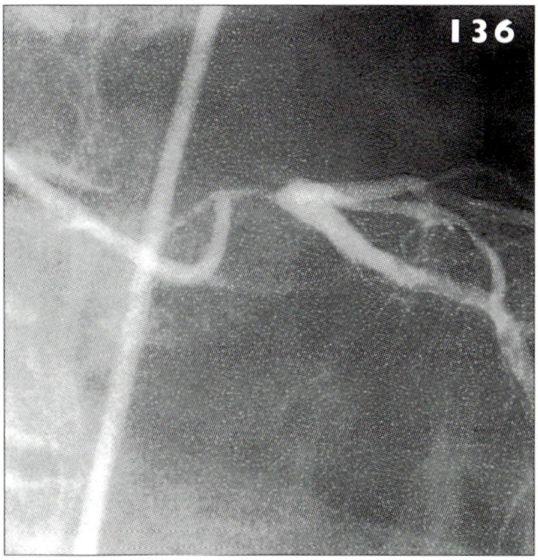

134 This man was driving his car and swerved to the left to avoid an on-coming vehicle. The other vehicle collided with him and his right forearm and sternum were fractured. However, in addition, he sustained a traumatic ventricular septal defect (visible near the cardiac apex), as can be seen on the angiogram. During left ventricular injection, contrast flows freely into the right ventricular chamber. Cardiac injury in trauma victims is common and demonstrable in up to 75% of fatalities; of cases of lethal traumatic injury to the heart, 5% have an acquired ventricular septal defect. Backwards movement of the sternum typically causes contusion of the anterior part of the heart. Sudden compression of the heart between the sternum and vertebral column is likely to be responsible for valvar and heart-wall damage, due to the abrupt rise in intraluminal pressure. From the point of view of treatment, the ventricular septal defect must be judged on its own merits. Thus, a small defect of little or no haemodynamic consequence and without appreciable left-to-right shunting can be left, whereas a larger lesion warrants urgent surgical repair.

135 The PR interval is prolonged to just above 0.3 s (normal range, 0.12–0.21 s). There are ST segment changes in leads I, aVl, V5 and V6, as well as T wave inversion in leads I and aVl. Prolongation of the PR interval characterises first-degree atrioventricular block – it represents delayed conduction through the atrioventricular junction. The abnormality is not associated with any symptoms. In young people it is usually due to high vagal tone and is benign. In older patients it may be caused by ischaemic heart disease, cardiac conduction tissue disease, or drugs causing delay of conduction at the atrioventricular node, such as beta-blockers, digoxin and certain calcium channel antagonists. The ST and T wave abnormalities seen in this ECG are probably non-specific, but may represent myocardial ischaemia or early cardiac conduction tissue disease. In the latter case some patients go on to develop higher degrees of atrioventricular block, which can be symptomatic or even life-threatening. These patients require permanent pacemaker implantation. (See also **44**.)

136 **i.** The angiogram shows a severe stenosis of the left main coronary artery. This is occasionally associated with breathlessness on exertion (usually with substantial ST segment depression on the exercise ECG) in the absence of angina pectoris.
ii. Left main stem disease is one of the presentations of coronary artery disease in which coronary bypass surgery is beneficial on prognostic as well as symptomatic grounds. The incidence of left main stem stenosis varies from 6–13% of patients with coronary disease and has a higher incidence in older patients (over the age of 70 years). There is also a higher incidence in those with a previous myocardial infarction, multiple cardiovascular risk factors, or a carotid bruit. Patients with angina at rest, low effort tolerance, or who experience recurrent pulmonary oedema should also be suspected of left main stem stenosis. Such patients often have resting ECG abnormalities and positive exercise tests at low workload.

137 A 53-year-old man with moderate-to-severe intermittent claudication was found to be hypertensive (blood pressure, 175/100 mmHg). He was commenced on captopril at a dose of 25 mg t.d.s., but this had little effect on the blood pressure. Overall, the patient felt worse, being particularly fatigued and nauseated.
i. What is the investigation shown?
ii. Give the underlying diagnosis and explain the clinical course.
iii. What is the incidence of this complication in the clinical context originally described?

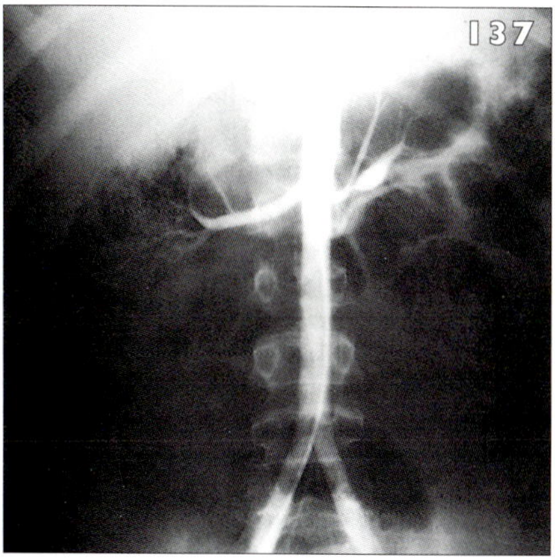

138 This valve comes from a 62-year-old woman whose predominant symptom over the previous 6 years had been breathlessness on exertion.
i. What is the diagnosis?
ii. Suggest an approximate valve area.
iii. List the haemodynamic findings which you might expect to find on invasive investigation.

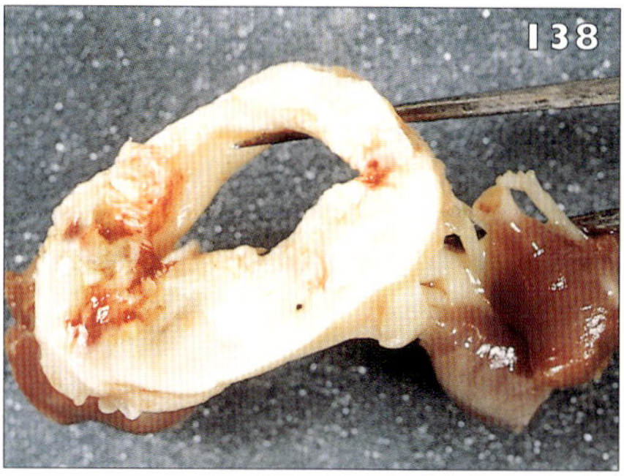

139 **i.** What is this?
ii. What are the indications for its use?

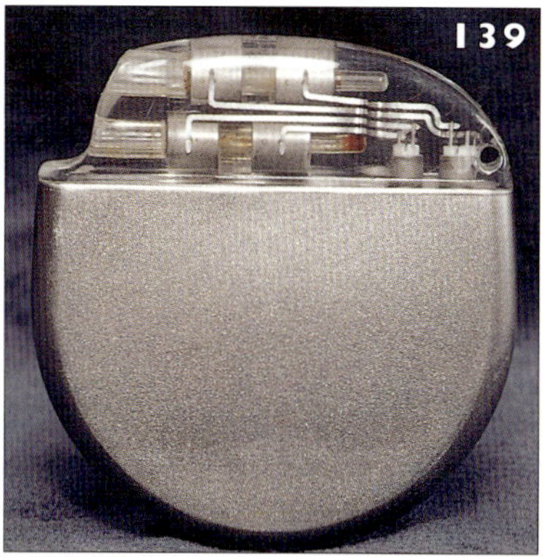

137 i. The investigation shown is a renal arteriogram.
ii. There is a stenosis of the left renal artery about 2 cm from the artery's origin, which is the cause of the patient's hypertension. Since he suffered from peripheral arterial disease, the renal artery stenosis is likely to be atheromatous rather than fibroelastic. In circumstances of renal artery stenosis, plasma renin and angiotensin levels are elevated. Administration of an angiotensin converting enzyme inhibitor results in dilatation of the efferent arterioles and a reduction in the effective filtration pressure across the glomerulus, with a concomitant worsening of renal function. In this case, the decline in renal function was symptomatic.
iii. Renal artery stenosis is common in the context of more generalised arteriopathy. It has a prevalence of about 20%.

138 i. An excised, stenosed mitral valve is shown (two leaflets can be defined). The combination of breathlessness on exertion and this gross pathological finding makes the clinical diagnosis mitral stenosis.
ii. The normal mitral valve area is about 4 cm^2. That of a significantly stenosed mitral valve is below 1 cm^2.
iii. The expecte haemodynamic findings would be:
(a) A pressure gradient across the mitral valve.
(b) Raised left atrial pressure.
(c) Raised pulmonary capillary wedge and arterial pressures.
(d) (Subsequently) raised right ventricular pressure and volume producing tricuspid regurgitation and elevated venous pressures.

139 i. This is a permanent pacemaker.
ii. Permanent pacing is used to treat symptomatic and life-threatening bradyarrhythmias. It is a very effective form of treatment and is now widely employeed in the management of the sick sinus syndrome, second- or third-degree atrioventricular block with or without atrial fibrillation, and carotid and vasovagal syndromes. Untreated third-degree atrioventricular block has a poor prognosis and carries a mortality approaching 30% per year. Treatment with cardiac pacing restores life expectancy to normal. Pacing in the sick sinus syndrome is associated with symptomatic benefit, but the prognosis is not altered. The effect of pacing in carotid and vasovagal syndromes depends upon the extent to which cardioinhibition contributes to the symptoms. In patients where the main cause of symptoms is the vasodilator mechanism, pacing is less effective.

Single and dual chamber pacemakers are available. Single chamber atrial stimulation is recommended in pure sick sinus syndrome where there is no evidence of atrioventricular block. Single chamber ventricular stimulation is recommended in patients with atrial fibrillation and atrioventricular block. All other conditions mentioned above should have dual atrial and ventricular pacemaker implants to prevent symptoms secondary to loss of atrial transport.

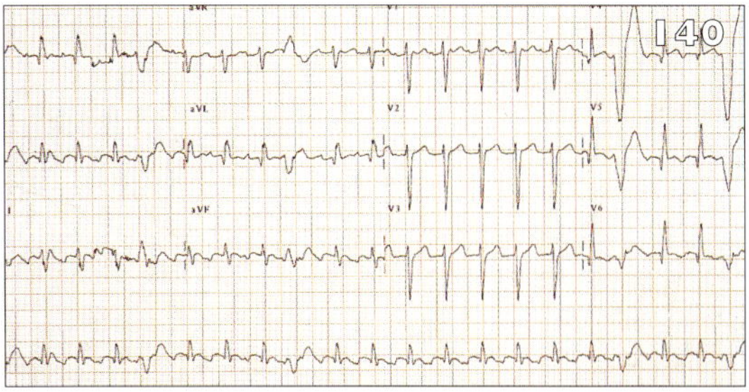

140 A 60-year-old man had suffered a myocardial infarction 6 months previously. On review in the clinic, although significantly limited in his effort tolerance, he said he felt reasonably well apart from an occasional fluttering in the throat. His ECG is shown.

i. What abnormality or abnormalities can you see?
ii. What is the prognostic significance of (**i**) in this context?
iii. How would you treat this patient?
iv. What are the risks inherent in your answer to (**iii**)?

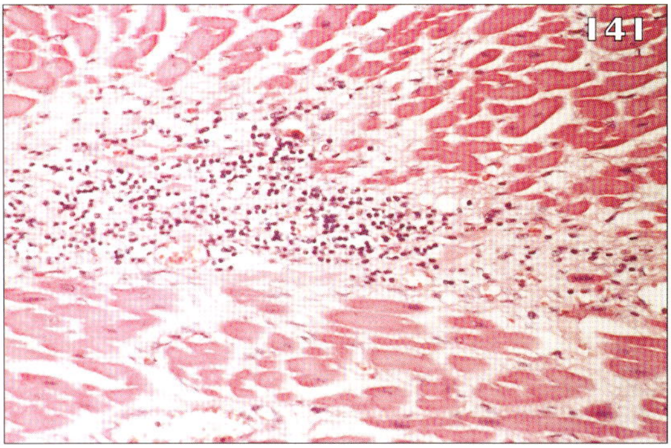

141 This was obtained from a mildly pyrexial 56-year-old man who had undergone cardiac transplantation 4 weeks before. What can you conclude?

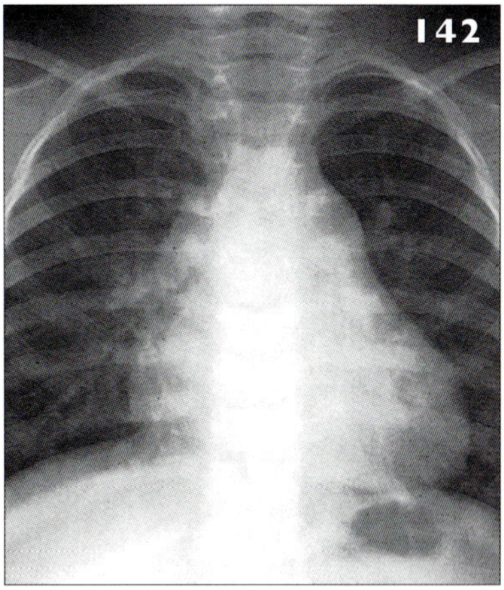

142 This 9-year-old girl had a murmur noted in early childhood. She had become increasingly breathless during the past year and was sometimes noted to look a bit blue.

i. Make two observations from the radiograph.
ii. Give the diagnosis.

140 i. The ECG shows frequent left ventricular premature beats (VPBs), with varying morphology.
ii. After acute myocardial infarction, the presence of frequent VPBs (>10/hour) carries an increased risk of sudden cardiac death, independent of the increase in risk due to impairment of left ventricular function. As well as this, complex forms of the VPBs, e.g. multiform or repetitive VPBs, bigeminy or short coupling intervals (approaching the R on T situation), add to the risk. VPBs after myocardial infarction have been classified by Lown: Grade 0 – no VPBs; Grade 1 – occasional VPBs (<30/hour); Grade 2 – frequent VPBs (>30/hour); Grade 3 – multiform VPBs; Grade 4a – couplets; Grade 4b – repetitive VPBs (3 or more); Grade 5 – R on T pattern of VPBs.
iii. Effective drugs include beta-blockers (which have the added benefit of post-infarction prophylaxis), the Class I agents disopyramide (1a), mexiletine (1b), and propafenone (1c), as well as the class III drug amiodarone. Ideally, the choice of drug would be made in conjunction with Holter monitoring (or an electrophysiological study if indicated).
iv. In the light of the Cardiac Arrhythmia Suppression Trial (CAST), many practitioners have formed the view that drugs are not indicated for the treatment of VPBs, unless they are causing symptoms or are so frequent that they there is haemodynamic compromise. Although the CAST study employed encainide and flecainide, there is no reason to believe that other anti-arrhythmic drugs would be safer. VPBs are associated with poor left ventricular function, which per se carries a poor prognosis. After suppression of the VPBs, the prognosis is still bad.

141 Endomyocardial biopsy remains the most reliable and most often employed technique for the detection (or confirmation) of cardiac allograft rejection. Microscopy shows the essential feature of diffuse myocardial interstitial (as well as perivascular) infiltration with mononuclear cells. In addition to this, myocyte necrosis is evident. This combination is characteristic of moderate acute rejection. In contrast, in mild acute rejection, the degree of interstitial infiltration is sparse and myocyte necrosis unusual. In severe acute rejection, interstitial infiltration is widespread and includes a wide range of cells (i.e. neutrophils and eosinophils, as well as lymphocytes), along with appreciable myocyte necrosis, haemorrhage, and even vasculitis.

142 i. The murmur noted in this girl's childhood was due to a ventricular septal defect of moderate size with obligatory pulmonary hypertension at the systemic level. She owed her survival to an increase in pulmonary vascular resistance which had prevented flooding of the lungs in infancy. The increase in right ventricular afterload caused right ventricular hypertrophy and enlargement, 'lifting' the left ventricular apex and producing the boot-shaped heart silhouette shown. The aortic knuckle is characteristically small. It is the high peripheral resistance of the pulmonary circulation, which reduces blood flow through the peripheral lung vasculature, that gives its 'pruned' appearance. Initially, this produces shunt reversal (and therefore cyanosis) only during exercise, but subsequently it is a constant feature.

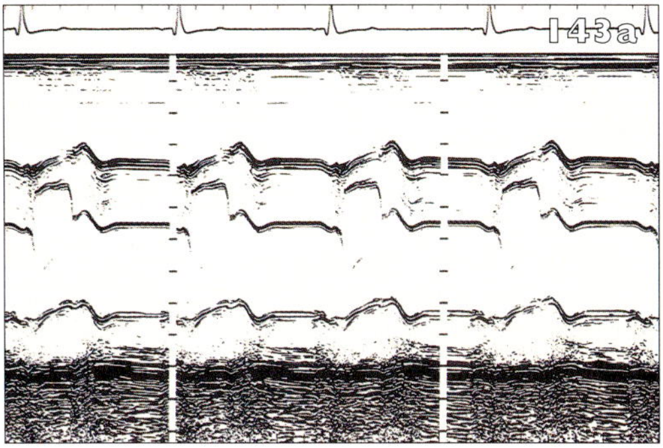

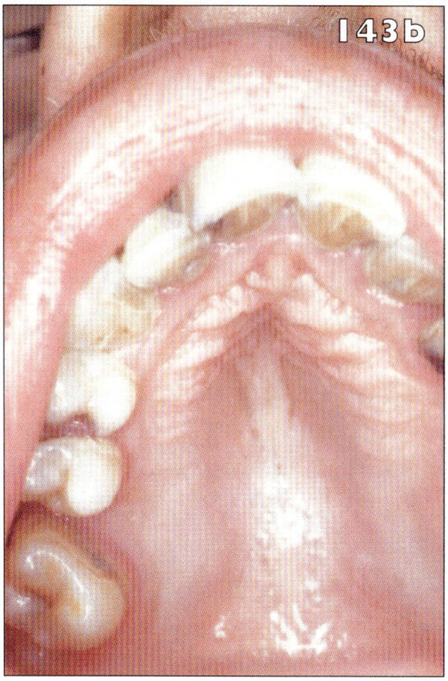

143 **i.** What is the investigation shown in **143a** and what does it show?
ii. What is shown in **143b**?
iii. Can you relate **143a** to **143b**?

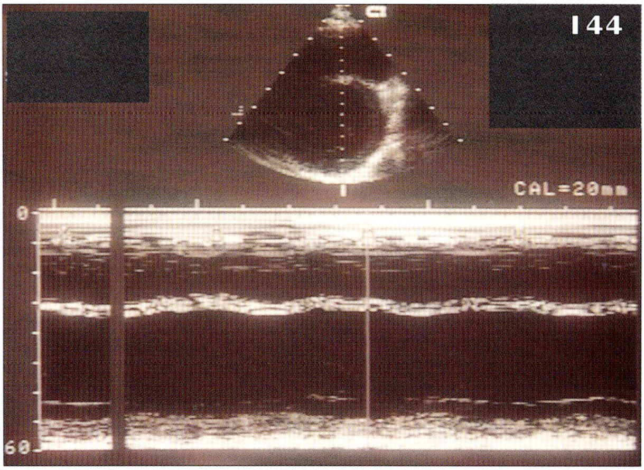

144 This is an M mode echocardiogram of a single 37-year-old male who had presented to his local hospital with arthritis 1 year earlier and was seen in the out-patient clinic complaining of breathlessness on exertion. On examination he had a low grade fever, oral candidiasis, and herpetic vesicles around the mouth. His heart rate was 120 b.p.m., his JVP was elevated, and auscultation of the heart revealed a loud third heart sound.
i. What is the abnormality?
ii. What is the probable underlying cause of this abnormality?

143 i. 143a is an M mode echocardiogram, the main feature of which is an abnormally wide aortic root.
ii. 143b shows a mouth with a high arched palate.
iii. The two features are related in Marfan's syndrome. This is a relatively common (10/100,000) autosomal dominant inherited disorder, characterised by abnormalities of the connective tissue component elastin. The disorder affects the skeleton, producing the typical phenotype of a tall subject with long extremities and digits (arachnodactyly) and the high arched palate shown. The consequences for the heart are a very high (>80%) rate of mitral valve prolapse [with obvious redundant tissue on the valve leaflets and an appreciable (ca. 25%) rate of significant mitral regurgitation] and dilatation of the sinuses of Valsalva and aortic root with regurgitation of the aortic valve. It is the latter which is the most significant feature, since dilatation of the aorta is associated with risk of acute aortic dissection (especially at aortic diameters >60 mm). The success rates of both elective and emergency aortic root reconstruction are very good. Unfortunately, prediction is difficult – e.g. Marfan aortas may dissect at 4.0 or 5.0 cm width. Family history is an important guide to prognosis.

144 i. The M mode is taken through the ventricular level and reveals a dilated, poorly contracting left ventricle. The normal range for left ventricular end-systolic dimension is 2.5–4.1 cm. The normal range for left ventricular end-diastolic dimension is 3.5–5.6 cm. Both systolic and diastolic dimensions are enlarged in this case. The ventricular septum and the posterior ventricular wall motion are significantly impaired.
ii. In a patient with previous sexually transmitted disease and evidence of current opportunistic infection the likely diagnosis is cardiomyopathy secondary to human immunodeficiency virus (HIV) infection. HIV cardiomyopathy is responsible for 7% of deaths from HIV infection – it manifests as global left ventricular dysfunction and occurs in the later stages of HIV infection. The signs and symptoms are those of congestive heart failure. Clinical characteristics associated with severe symptomatic cardiac dysfunction include low CD4 T cell counts and persistent elevation of anti-heart antibodies. The latter suggests that cardiac autoimmunity may play a role in the pathogenesis of HIV cardiomyopathy. Treatment is as for dilated cardiomyopathy. Other cardiac manifestations of HIV include non-bacterial thrombotic endocarditis, infectious and serous pericardial effusions, myocarditis secondary to opportunistic organisms, and cardiac neoplasms, such as lymphoma or Kaposi's sarcoma.

145 This 39-year-old woman with a 6-month history of increasing breathlessness and joint pains had been treated in hospital for declining renal function. After a few days, she felt worse and was noted to have a pyrexia of 38.5°C and a late systolic murmur.
i. What is the underlying disease?
ii. Give an explanation of the events described.

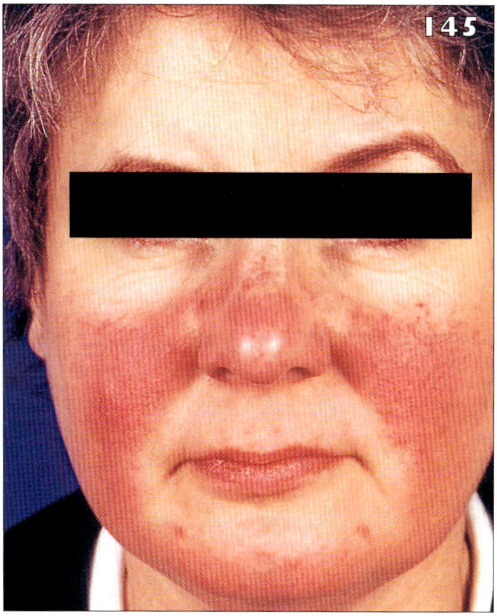

146 A 62-year-old woman presented with three transient episodes of collapse within 24 hours. She had recently been noted to have hypertension and had been commenced on a thiazide diuretic. An ECG was taken in the emergency department while the patient was asymptomatic.
i. What are the abnormalities on the ECG?
ii. Suggest a possible aetiological factor.

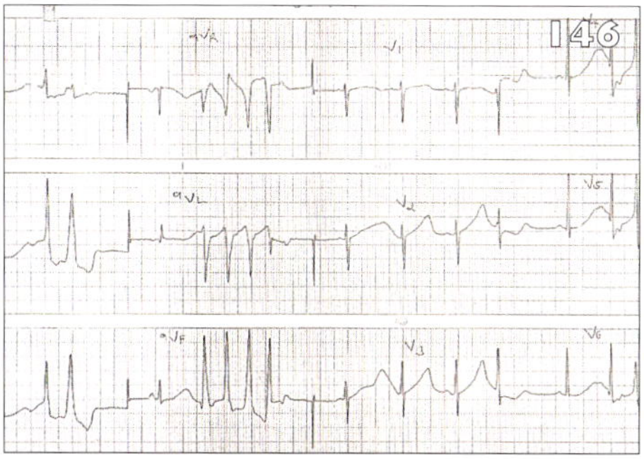

147 What was the cause of death in this man said to have had an 'irregular pulse' when routinely examined 3 weeks previously?

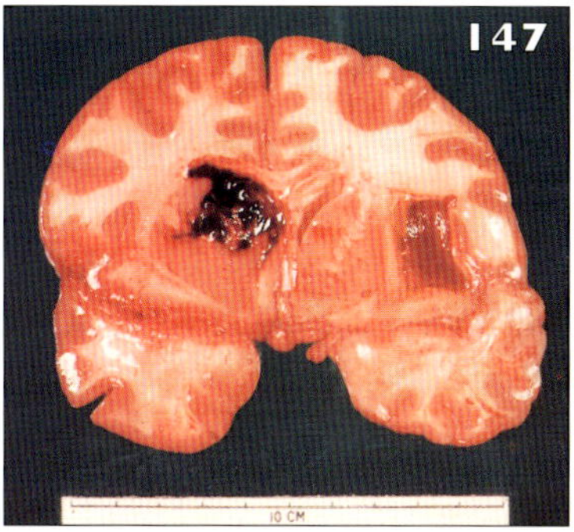

145 i. The woman has erythema on the cheeks and across the bridge of her nose in the classical 'butterfly' distribution, which is characteristic of systemic lupus erythematosus (SLE); it is present in about 80% of cases of SLE.
ii. The 6-month history of increasing breathlessness, joint pains and decline in renal function all point to an aggressive course of the disease, which is being treated with both steroids and immunosuppressant steroid-sparing drugs. The development of a late systolic murmur suggests the occurrence of mitral regurgitation. This may be due to Libman–Sacks endocarditis, a direct complication of SLE, or, as she has become febrile, to infective endocarditis, an unfortunate complication mostly attributable to the treatment for SLE. Libman–Sacks endocarditis was described as a classic feature of SLE, but although found in about 10% of autopsy cases, it is not especially common clinically. One or more verrucose lesions usually occur on the mitral and (less commonly) aortic valve leaflets with underlying fibrosis. In the case in question, the pyrexia and treatment suggest infective endocarditis in an immunosuppressed subject as the more likely diagnosis of the two. Blood cultures are needed, followed by antibiotics; fever due to infection responds to antibiotics, but fever due to autoimmune disease does not.

146 i. The ECG reveals short runs of polymorphic ventricular tachycardia and a long Q-T interval. The Q-T interval in this case measures 0.52 s (normal corrected Q-T interval is 0.44 s). Prolongation of the Q-T interval predisposes to polymorphic ventricular tachycardia, which is usually not sustained but can degenerate into ventricular fibrillation. The transient losses of consciousness in this patient were probably secondary to periods of ventricular tachycardia longer than those seen on the ECG.
ii. The most likely predisposing factor is hypokalaemia secondary to the thiazide diuretic. Other electrolyte abnormalities that lead to prolongation of the Q-T interval include hypocalcaemia and hypomagnesaemia. Management in this case involves reducing the Q-T interval by increasing the heart rate while trying to correct the electrolyte abnormality. This would require either atrial pacing at a rate exceeding 60 b.p.m or using intravenous isoprenaline to produce the same effect (see also **218**).

147 This question highlights the answer to **77iii**. The man in question had paroxysmal atrial fibrillation, hence the irregular pulse. In this case there was also underlying undiagnosed mitral stenosis, a combination that is associated with a high risk of embolic stroke. Thus, while there is a five-fold increase in stroke incidence in cases of untreated 'lone' atrial fibrillation, the increased incidence in post-rheumatic valve disease is more like seventeen-fold. A cerebral infarct is shown, which was the immediate cause of death in this patient.

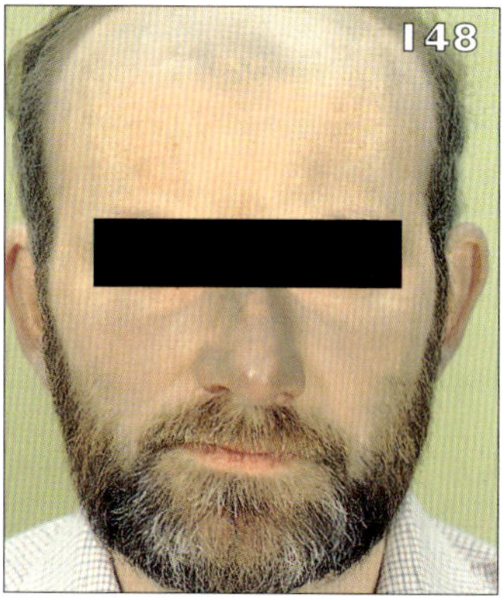

148 This patient was started on medical therapy for palpitations (frequent 'dropped beats') subsequent to an acute myocardial infarction. On further questioning, the only other complaint was one of recent-onset impotence and testicular discomfort.

i. What was the drug?

ii. Predict the likely values for testosterone, follicle stimulating hormone (FSH), and luteinising hormone (LH) in this patient.

iii. What is the outlook on stopping the therapy?

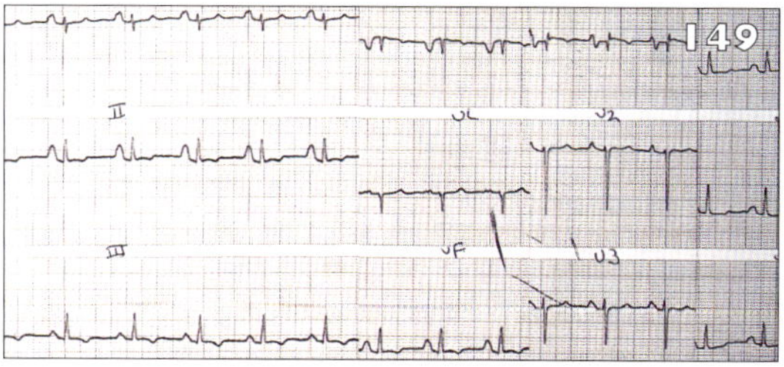

149 A 55-year-old retired naval engineer complained to his family doctor of a worsening breathlessness on exertion. The family doctor noted central cyanosis and heard an expiratory wheeze on auscultation of the chest.

i. What is the most likely diagnosis?

ii. How would you confirm your opinion?

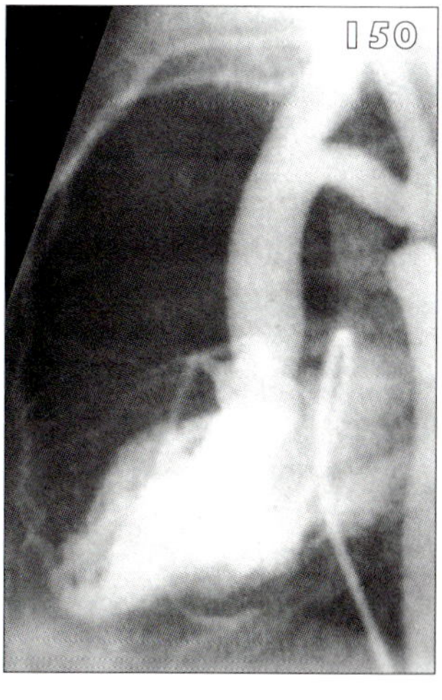

150 A 35-year-old hypertensive man underwent an investigation.

i. What is this investigation?

ii. What is the diagnosis?

148 i. This patient had severe three-vessel coronary artery disease, but for a number of reasons a medical course of management was pursued. One component of the drug regimen was amiodarone, since the man had frequent ventricular premature beats – he has a typical slate-grey amiodarone skin discoloration. This can persist for years after cessation of the drug, but it does gradually fade.
ii. A rare side effect of amiodarone therapy is epididymo-orchitis. This patient kept quiet about testicular discomfort and, later on, about becoming impotent for several months. Primary testicular failure developed, so testosterone (normally produced in the testis) will be reduced, but FSH and LH will be raised due to lack of feedback inhibition from the testis to the anterior pituitary (testosterone and inhibin).
iii. The outlook largely depends on how long the therapy has been used. Generally, once the problem has developed, the outlook for recovery of testicular function is poor.

149 i. This 55-year-old ex-sailor had smoked 20 cigarettes a day for many years and developed cor pulmonale secondary to chronic obstructive airways disease. The effect of loss of lung tissue and pulmonary vascular constriction (probably due to hypoxia) is to cause pulmonary hypertension (see **226**). Alveolar hypoventilation with carbon dioxide retention and hypoxaemia ensue and lead to fluid retention. There is a rise in systemic venous pressure, with associated signs of right heart failure. On examination of this patient, there were signs suggestive of type II respiratory failure (see also **9**). On the ECG, note the right ventricular hypertrophy, right atrial enlargement and right axis deviation, as well as the reduced size of the complexes.
ii. Further investigations of value include arterial blood gases (which show the low P_aO_2 and elevated P_aCO_2 of Type II respiratory failure), lung function tests (which may show airflow limitation – i.e. reduced FEV_1, FVC, and the ratio FEV_1/FVC ; lung volumes normal or increased; transfer factor, K_{CO}, low, reflecting the loss of functioning lung tissue), and tests for both haemoglobin and packed cell volume, which are typically elevated (secondary polycythaemia due to hypoxia). The chest radiograph may show bullae, reduced peripheral lung markings and flat diaphragms with cardiomegaly.

150 i. This is an aortic angiogram, which shows a stenosis of the descending aorta. There is hypoplasia at the site of the obstruction and post-stenotic dilatation.
ii. The patient has coarctation of the aorta, a relatively common congenital heart lesion found in about 1/4000 live births, more commonly among males. It is frequent in Turner's syndrome. The diagnosis should be made in infancy or young childhood, but occasionally patients still present with hypertension in adulthood. The upper limb hypertension is accompanied by a decreased pulse pressure below the coarctation and radial–femoral arterial pulse delay may be detected clinically. In addition to the straightforward radiological appearances, the fact that the condition was not detected until adulthood also argues against the lesion being anything other than an isolated coarctation, since complex lesions (e.g. with patency of the arterial duct or an associated ventricular septal defect) present much earlier, often with congestive cardiac failure in infancy or childhood.

151 A 60-year-old woman from the Indian subcontinent was admitted with increasing ankle swelling. She had suffered from tuberculosis at the age of 31. On examination she was tachypnoeic, her heart rate was 105 b.p.m., blood pressure 90/70 mmHg, JVP elevated 8 cm above the sternal angle and the respiratory rate was 20/min. Her heart sounds were quiet and chest was clear, but her abdomen was grossly distended and shifting dullness was demonstrable. There was evidence of considerable lower limb oedema.
Investigations are on the right.
i. What is the most likely diagnosis?
ii. List one non-invasive and one invasive test you would request prior to commencing treatment.

Full blood count

Haemoglobin	13 g/dl
Bilirubin	20 mmol/l
WCC	4.2 x 10^9/l
AST	21 IU/l
Platelets	300 x 10^9/l
Albumin	40 g/l

Biochemistry

Sodium	133 mmol/l
Potassium	5.0 mmol/l
Urea	9 mmol/l
(BUN	25.2 mg/dl)
Creatinine	104 µmol/l (1.18 mg/dl)

Chest radiograph

Gross cardiomegaly, evidence of scarring in the right upper lobe.

152 The 50-year-old patient whose hands are shown here had a 'murmur' noticed during a routine medical some years ago. As she had no symptoms, apart from fatigue on moderate exertion (which she put down to being out of condition and overworked), the woman defaulted from follow-up. Her symptoms worsened over about 18 months and her hands changed to the above.
i. What physical sign is shown?
ii. Suggest three causes.

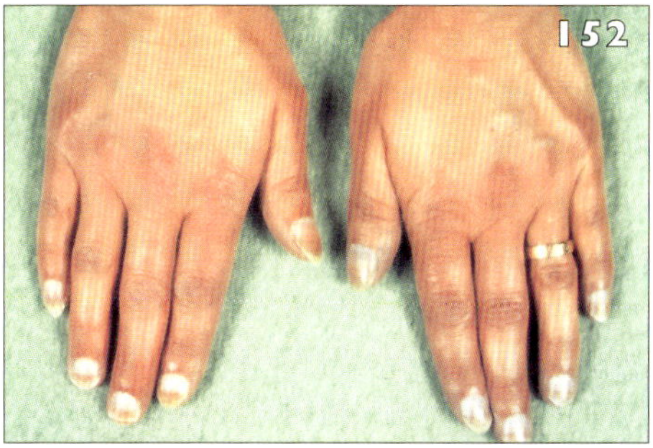

153 This ECG (**153a**) was obtained from an asymptomatic 37-year-old woman. What does it show?

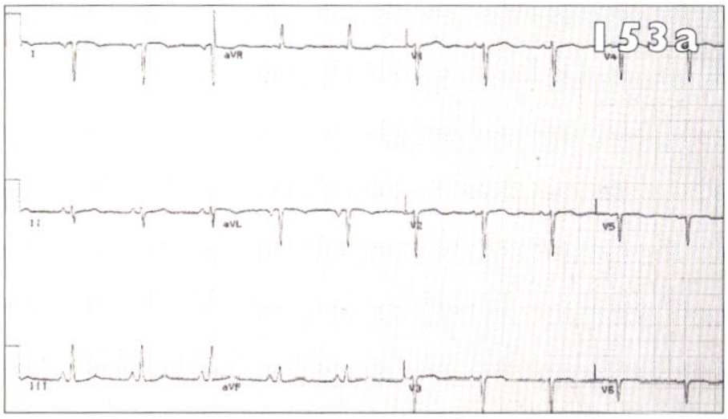

151 i. The chest radiograph report describes cardiomegaly, which is probably due to a pericardial effusion secondary to tuberculosis.
ii. Echocardiography is the non-invasive test; the invasive test would be pericardiocentesis with pericardial fluid drainage and sampling for protein content, bacteriology (including acid-fast bacilli) and cytology. Tuberculous pericarditis usually follows the spread of infection from adjacent mediastinal lymph nodes. Pericardial effusion may be the presenting feature of tuberculous infection. Early symptoms of pericarditic symptoms may have been present for several weeks, as well as malaise and night sweats – cardiac tamponade is common. Constrictive pericarditis is likely to follow. The diagnostic yield from pericardial fluid culture is approximately 25%. Surgical biopsy of the pericardium followed by histology and culture of the specimen is more likely to be diagnostic. Anti-tuberculous therapy is required and should be continued for one year.

152 i. The physical sign is clubbing of the fingers.
ii. Clubbing of the digits is associated with cyanotic heart disease, suppurative lung disease, carcinoma of the lung, fibrosing alveolitis, infective endocarditis and biliary cirrhosis. It is also found as a benign familial trait. In the context of this question, three possible causes would be a congenital heart lesion with shunt reversal due to the progression of pulmonary vascular disease, a slow-growing squamous carcinoma of the lung, or pulmonary arteriovenous fistula (usually associated with hereditary telangiectasia).

153 The gradual reduction in QRS size from V1 to V6, the negative P and QRS in I, and the positive P and QRS in aVR make dextrocardia the obvious diagnosis. The chest radiograph (**153b**) confirms this, provided careful attention is paid to the labelling of it! From the radiograph, it can be seen that the gastric air bubble is on the same side as the cardiac apex, i.e. there is situs inversus rather than an isolated dextrocardia. Clinically, dextrocardia can often be diagnosed by palpation of the cardiac apex on the right side of the thorax. A minority of cases of congenital dextrocardia are also associated with basal bronchiectasis, infection of the cranial sinuses, and malformation of the frontal sinuses, i.e. Kartagener's syndrome. Isolated dextrocardia (laevocardia) is associated with complex congenital heart disease. Perhaps unsurprisingly, dextrocardia is also associated with left handedness.

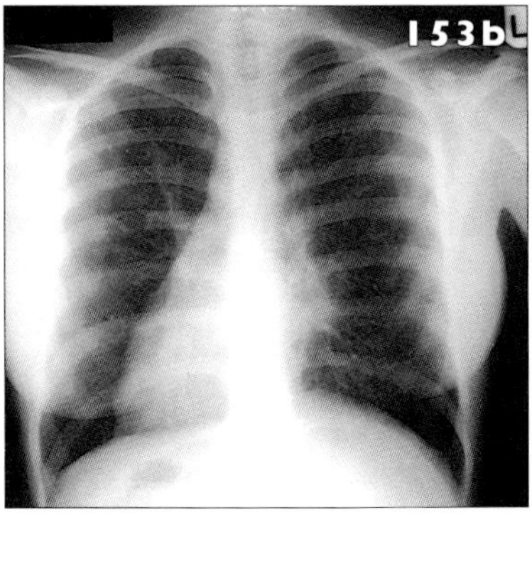

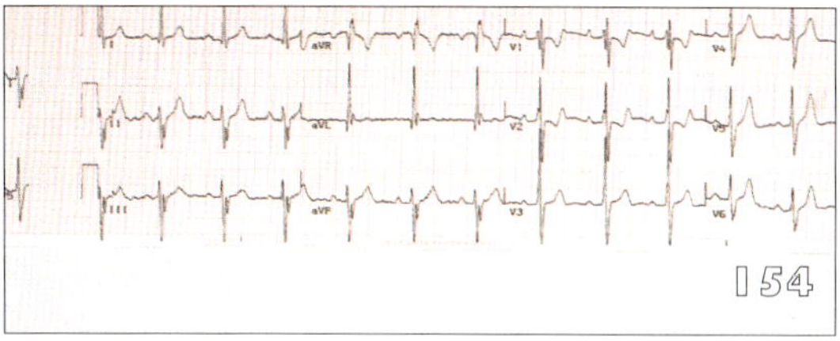

154

154 A 23-year-old Somali woman was referred to a local cardiologist at 30 weeks' gestation because she was noted to have had a cardiac murmur at a very young age. She had recently emigrated from Somalia and could not reliably give further details about the murmur. As a child she had experienced recurrent respiratory tract infections and was not keen on sports activities because she tired easily. This was her first pregnancy, which thus far had been uncomplicated. On examination she appeared well. There was no evidence of cyanosis or clubbing, heart rate was 90 b.p.m. and regular, and blood pressure was normal. On examination of the precordium the apex was thrusting and there was a palpable right ventricular heave. Auscultation revealed a loud pan-systolic murmur in the mitral area and a softer ejection systolic murmur in the pulmonary area. The pulmonary component to the second heart sound was loud.

i. List two abnormalities on the ECG.

ii. What is the diagnosis?

iii. How would you account for the murmur in the mitral area?

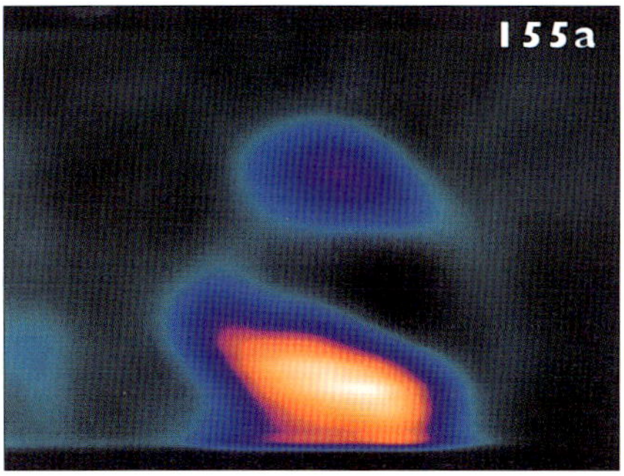

155a

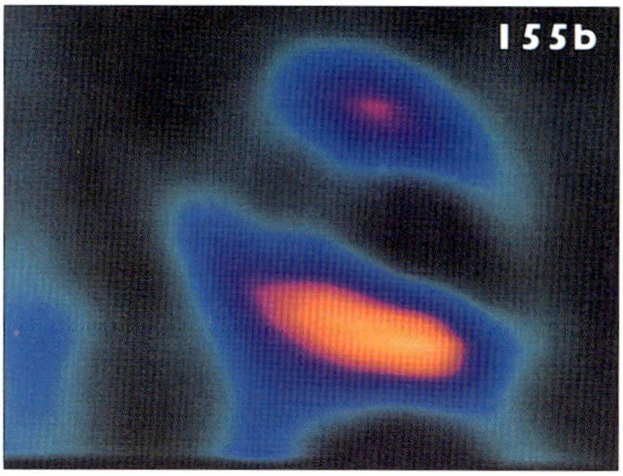

155b

155 A 67-year-old male patient with a fairly typical history of effort-related angina and left bundle branch block (LBBB) on the resting ECG was referred for further investigation and a procedure was carried out, the results being shown here. **155a** was taken at time zero and **155b** after 4 hours.

i. What is this investigation?

ii. What is its sensitivity and specificity in the detection of coronary artery disease?

iii. What conclusion is to be drawn from the test? Can a development of the technique give you more information?

154 i. Two abnormalities are that the axis is shifted to the left and there is evidence of partial right bundle branch block and deep S waves in leads V5 and V6.
ii. The history, physical examination, and ECG changes are consistent with the diagnosis of ostium primum atrial septal defect (partial atrioventricular canal).
iii. Ostium primum atrial septal defect is due to maldevelopment of the endocardial cushions. The anterior mitral valve leaflet is cleft and the valve is usually regurgitant. The defect is common in Down syndrome and is rarely associated with Klinefelter's and Noonan's syndromes. The ECG demonstrates a leftward axis in contrast to an ostium secundum defect, in which the axis is rightward. Right bundle branch block is common to both types of defect.

155 i. This is a single photon emission computed tomograph (SPECT) study with 201-thallium. Thallium is a cation which behaves like potassium and is distributed regionally within the heart according to the cardiac output. Thus, areas which are hypoperfused take up less tracer than well-perfused areas, so a relative defect appears on the image. If the defect is constant, i.e. present at rest and after myocardial stress, then the area is most likely scar tissue. However, if the defect is only present under stress conditions, then the area of myocardium in question is viable, but subtended by a coronary artery which is significantly stenosed. The difference between SPECT and planar thallium imaging is that the SPECT image acquisition is three-dimensional and therefore offers a much-improved spatial resolution.
ii. In a recent series, the sensitivity and specificity of myocardial perfusion scintigraphy in angiographically confirmed coronary artery disease were, respectively, 80% and 92%.
iii. In the case in question, the patient has a typical history of angina and LBBB on the resting ECG. The thallium scan shows an anteroapical perfusion defect (**155a**) persistent at 4 hours (**155b**). This may represent an area of myocardial scarring, but its localisation, combined with the LBBB, suggests significant disease in the territory of the left anterior descending (LAD) coronary artery. Repeat imaging later than 4 hours, with or without re-injection of thallium, is an important refinement of the technique. It may reveal late reversibility of the perfusion defect and hence viability of the particular area of myocardium.

156 Mr Smith, 26 years old, decided to have himself investigated for risk of cardiac disease after his 35-year-old brother had a myocardial infarction. Their father had died 15 years previously of a myocardial infarction. An electrophoretic strip for lipoprotein analysis is shown.
i. What is the diagnosis?
ii. What is its mode of inheritance?
iii. What are the implications for cardiovascular risk?

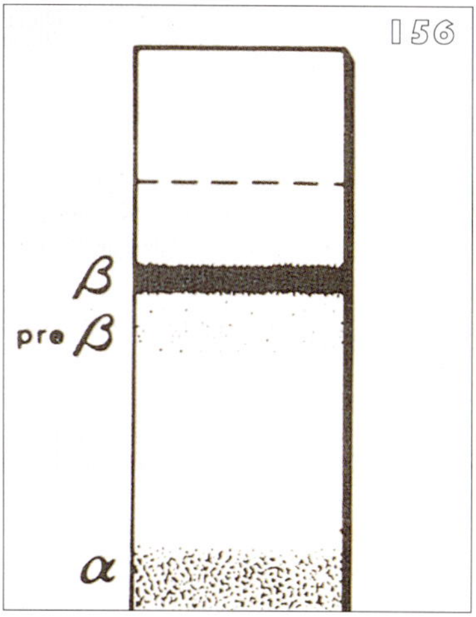

157 As you approach the cardiology outpatient clinic, you notice that this little girl is waiting to be seen with her mother. Without any prior knowledge about this particular girl, what cardiovascular disorders might come to mind?

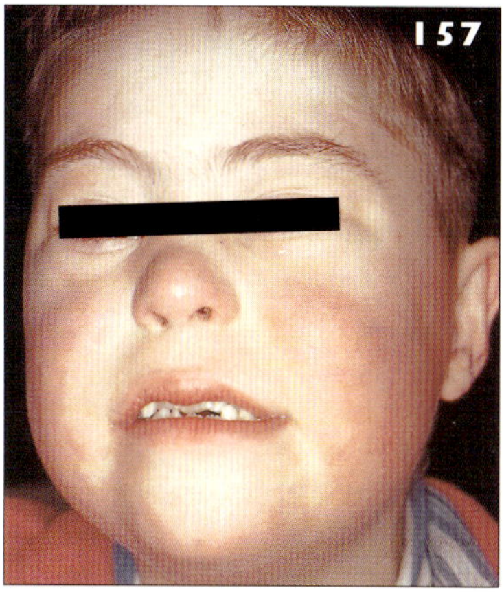

158 What can be deduced from these ECG rhythm strips?

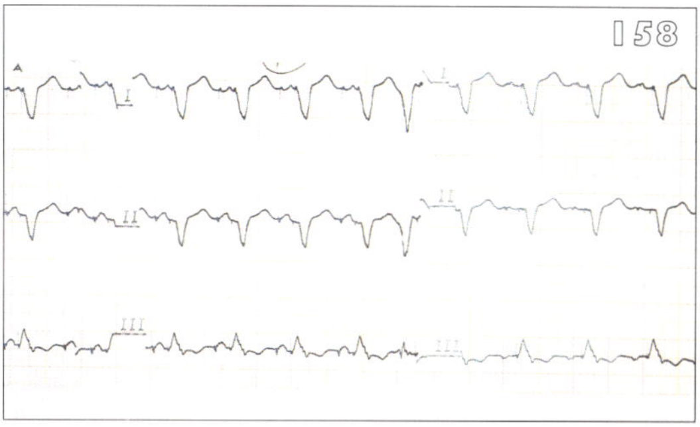

156 i. The electrophoretic strip shows an excess of low density lipoprotein (LDL, also known as β-lipoprotein) as the only biochemical lesion. The levels of very low density lipoprotein (VLDL, also known as pre-β-lipoprotein) and high density lipoprotein (HDL, also known as α-lipoprotein) are normal. The diagnosis, following the Frederickson classification, is Type IIa familial hypercholesterolaemia (FH).
ii. FH has a prevalence of about 0.2%. It is an autosomal dominantly inherited disorder due to a mutation of the gene coding for the LDL receptor.
iii. If homozygous, the disease may present in childhood with advanced coronary artery disease (CAD) or aortic stenosis. More commonly, it is the heterozygous form of the disease which is detected. In the latter, about 50% of males and 12% of females develop CAD by 50 years of age, and 85% of males and 60% of females by 60 years of age. This degree of CAD is found about 20 years later in a non-FH population. The relative risk of myocardial infarction is about ten times that of a non-FH population. Clinically, tendon xanthomata and xanthelasmata may be found in FH, as well as signs which reflect premature atheroma.

157 This girl has Down syndrome (trisomy of chromosome 21), a relatively common chromosomal abnormality, with an overall incidence of 1/800 births (significantly higher as the maternal age rises above 40). Since about 40% of children with Down syndrome have an associated congenital heart lesion, it is associated with 1 in 20 cardiac malformations. Of Down children with a cardiac abnormality, 40% have an isolated atrioventricular canal defect which is either growth or adhesion of the endocardial cushions. These are involved in the embryological division of the cardiac atria and ventricles. In complete defects, there is a common orifice between the atria and ventricles with confluent atrial and ventricular septal defects. The partial form of the abnormality, with separate right and left atrioventricular orifices, used to be called an ostium primum septal defect, but this is embryologically incorrect. The left atrioventricular valve has a cleft anterior leaflet and regurgitation may be mild or severe. Development of pulmonary hypertension and pulmonary vascular disease is particularly common in Down syndrome and determines the cardiovascular prognosis.

158 The ECG demonstrates dual chamber pacing. Pacing spikes precede most P waves and all the QRS complexes. In the last few complexes the patient's own P wave occurs before and therefore inhibits the atrial pacing spike. The P wave then triggers a ventricular impulse. Dual chamber pacing is used in bradyarrhythmias with normal atrial contraction, except in pure sick sinus syndrome when single chamber atrial pacing suffices. Dual chamber pacing has the advantage of maintaining atrial transport, which is effectively lost with single chamber ventricular stimulation.

159 In the course of investigating a 73-year-old man with chest pain, this image was obtained.
i. How would you describe this coronary artery?
ii. What is its pathological basis?

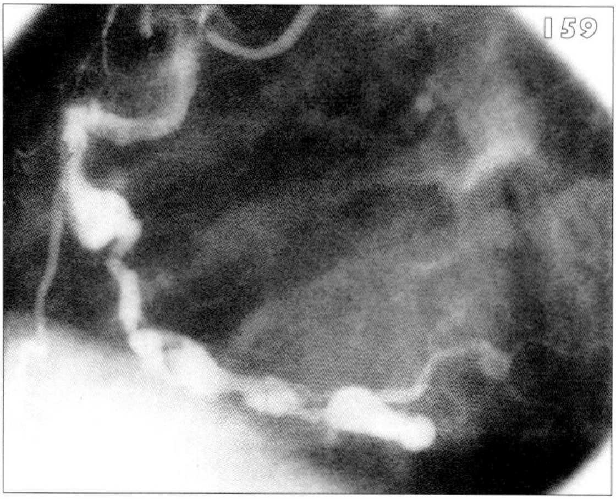

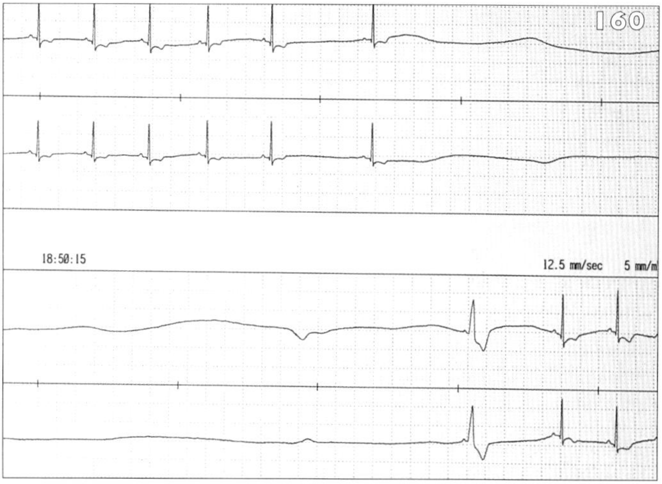

160 A 25-year-old man had complained of two episodes of collapse with loss of consciousness in 3 months. After a number of other investigations, he was reviewed at a tertiary referral centre and placed on a tilt table. After 20 minutes of head-up tilt, he suddenly lost consciousness and the ECG was as shown.
i. What does the ECG show?
ii. What is the underlying diagnosis?
iii. What treatment options are there for this young man?

159 This right coronary artery is ectatic. Ectasia of a coronary artery was defined in the Coronary Artery Surgery Study (CASS) as a vessel of diameter up to 1.5 times the diameter of the adjacent normal vessel. The incidence of the problem is a little less than 4% of patients with angina or coronary artery disease who undergo angiography. The right coronary artery is affected in most cases (75%).
ii. Coronary ectasia is commonly associated with stenotic disease; however, ischaemia and infarction have been reported in the territory of ectatic vessels, even in the absence of luminal stenosis. Coronary blood flow is slowed in coronary ectasia and a tendency to platelet aggregation and arterial thrombosis has been postulated. In addition, a predisposition to coronary spasm in response to ergonovine has been demonstrated. The slightly higher incidence in patients who also have abdominal aortic aneurysm and the similar microscopic histology of the two conditions has pointed to a common aetiology – atheroma. The external circumference of atheromatous vessels is increased, even though the lumen may be narrowed. In coronary ectasia, this dilatation is exaggerated.

160 i. The ECG shows a prolonged sinus pause. It is not possible on the basis of the ECG alone to discern the cause of the pause. Sinoatrial dysfunction would be a likely reason for this, but the rarer hypersensitive carotid sinus syndrome or vasovagal syndrome could also be causative.
ii. In the context of this particular case, the history of collapse as well as the tilt-table findings (which showed inducible syncope) are typical of 'malignant' vasovagal syncope. In this condition, which is essentially a disorder of central neural autonomic regulation of the circulation, intense vagal discharges lead to a combination of cardio-inhibition and peripheral vasodepression. Thus, hypotension combines with bradycardia to cause the fall in cerebral perfusion which manifests as syncope.
iii. The treatment of choice would be a dual chamber pacing system, although support stockings have been of value in some patients, as has oral propantheline, scopolamine patches (anticholinergic) and combinations of ephedrine and propranolol (producing a sympathetic α-vasoconstrictive action). Pacing is only effective by preventing bradycardia; if there is a marked vasodepressor element to the attacks, pacing will fail. Beta-blockers with strong partial agonist action, such as xamoterol, should be tried.

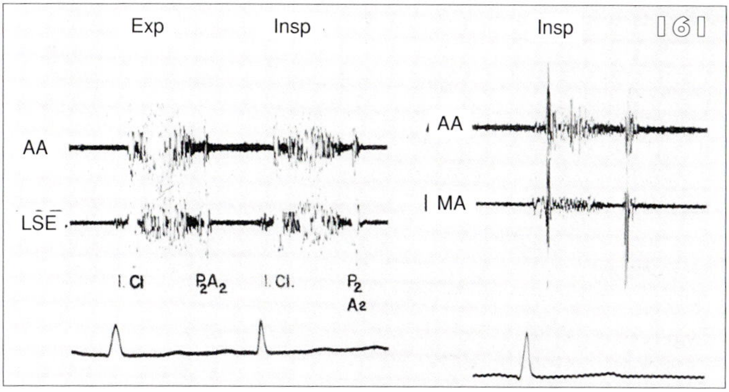

161 The tracers on the right are from a normal subject, while those on the left were obtained from a patient with echocardiographically demonstrated moderate aortic stenosis and left bundle branch block on the ECG.

What abnormalities can be seen on the phonocardiogram and how might these be discerned on physical examination? (AA, aortic area; LSE, left sternal edge; MA, mitral area; Exp, expiration; Ins, inspiration.)

162 In order further to investigate his angina, a 65-year-old man underwent cardiac catheterisation by Sones' method. During the injection which produced the image shown, the patient developed an acute pain in the chest.

i. What does the image show?

ii. What action should be taken?

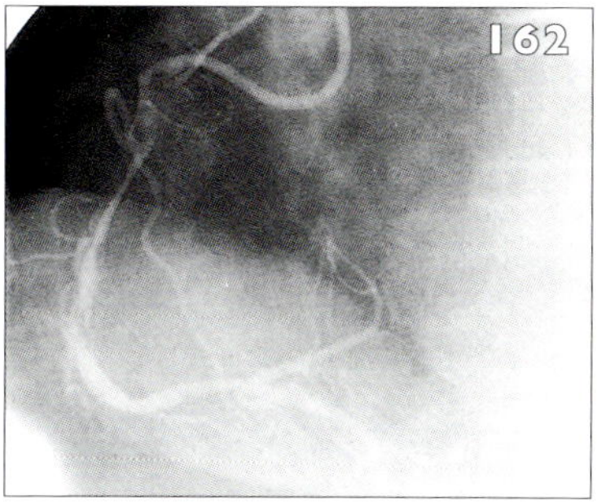

163 This man was breathless. What is the visible abnormality?

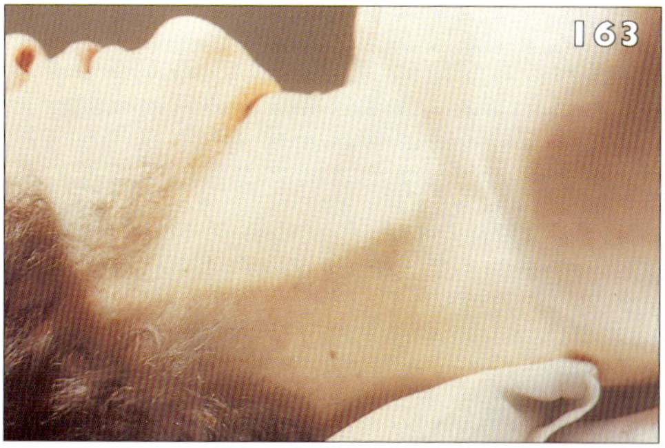

161 There is a crescendo–decrescendo systolic murmur visible on the phonocardiogram. In addition, there is reversed splitting of the second heart sound in this patient. The ECG showed left bundle branch block. In left bundle branch block, the delayed electrical activation of the left ventricle causes A2 to be delayed. Thus splitting of S2 is wider in expiration because P2 (which is normally delayed because of the increased right ventricular stroke volume during inspiration) is abnormally close to (or fuses with) the delayed A2. This phenomenon, a wider split of the aortic and pulmonary components of S2 during expiration, is known as reversed splitting of the second heart sound.

162 **i.** The angiogram shows an irregular spiralling opacification along the length of the right coronary artery. There has been a dissection of this vessel.
ii. This occurrence during a diagnostic angiogram can be disastrous – the situation is less frequently retrievable than if a dissection occurs during percutaneous angioplasty, with a guide wire already down the vessel lumen. Sometimes, if a balloon catheter can be positioned across the site of the dissection flap, a prolonged inflation can help to fix the flap down. If feasible, a coronary artery stent could be deployed. A perfusion balloon catheter would be of value to maintain distal coronary flow. Emergency coronary artery bypass grafting may or may not be necessary, depending on whether the dissection flap re-adheres or the artery occludes, whether or not the right coronary artery was dominant, and whether there are stenoses in the left coronary system which might require grafting.

163 The JVP is elevated. Elevated JVP occurs in congestive cardiac failure due to elevation of right ventricular pressure and the consequent elevation of right atrial pressure. There are no valves between the internal jugular vein and the right atrium, so the elevation of pressure is transmitted directly to the internal jugular vein and is visible on examining the neck. The JVP is also elevated in constrictive pericarditis, cardiac tamponade, volume overload and superior vena caval obstruction. In the last case venous pulsation is absent. In constrictive pericarditis and cardiac tamponade, right ventricular filling is increased during inspiration compared with left ventricular filling. The total cardiac filling does not increase, although the venous return to the thorax does and consequently venous pressure paradoxically increases during this phase of respiration – Kussmaul's sign. Large a waves are caused by an increase in resistance to right ventricular filling and are seen in pulmonary hypertension or pulmonary stenosis. Very large a waves occur in complete heart block and ventricular tachycardia, when the atria contract against a closed tricuspid valve. These large waves are commonly known as Cannon waves. Large v waves occur in tricuspid regurgitation.

164 A healthy 22-year-old woman volunteer was invited to breathe out against the constant pressure resistance of a mercury column. After 3 s the resistance was abolished. The traces show heart rate and blood pressure responses to this challenge.
i. Which trace is the true one for this woman?
ii. Explain the sequence of changes.

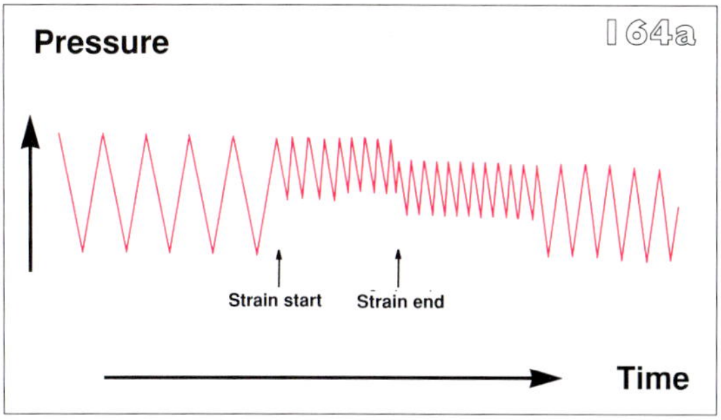

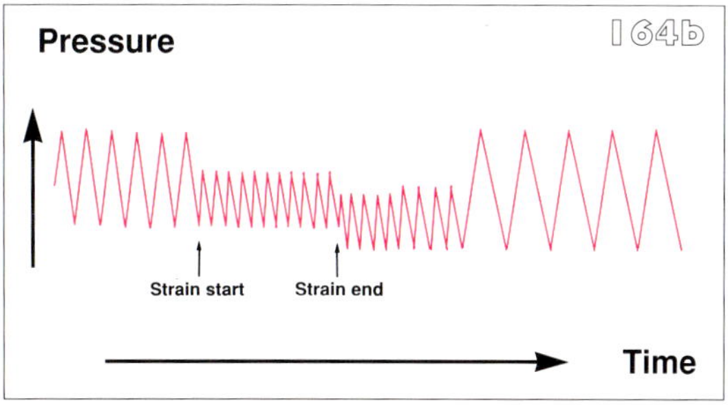

165 This post-mortem heart has been stained with potassium ferricyanide. What is the diagnosis?

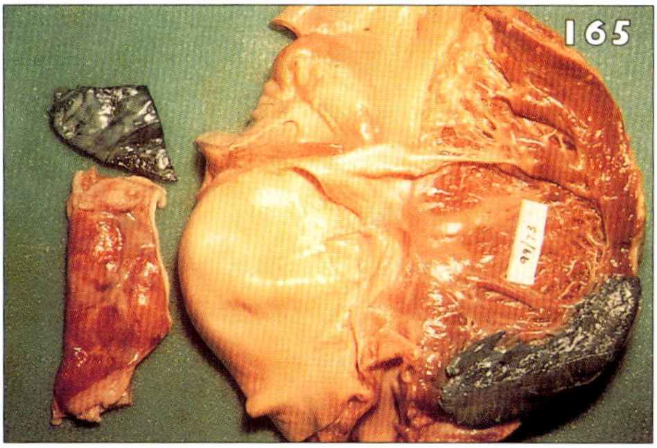

166 A 37-year-old bank employee was referred to out-patients complaining of 'palpitations'. The resting ECG was as shown.
i. What abnormalities can you see?
ii. Give five common causes for the problem.

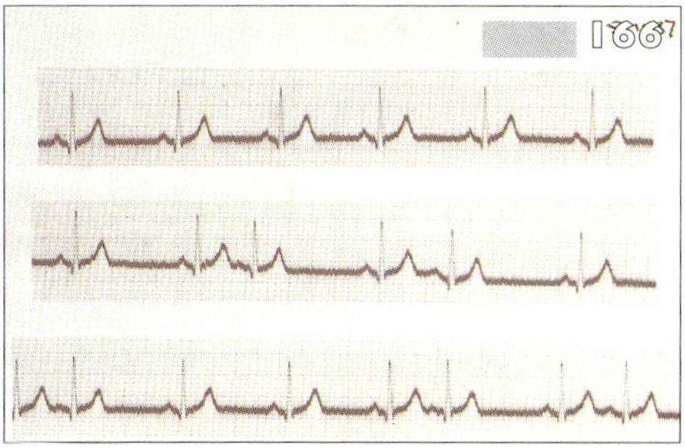

164 i. **164b** is the true representation of the Valsalva manoeuvre.
ii. The phases of the Valsalva manoeuvre are: Phase I: the increase in intrathoracic pressure caused by expiration against a closed glottis produces an initial rise in blood pressure. Phase II: an increase in heart rate with a reduction in both blood pressure and pulse pressure. Phase III: on release of the strain, blood pressure and pulse pressure fall further. Phase IV: a rise in blood pressure to above the resting level, accompanied by a slowing of the heart rate.
The above applies to healthy individuals. In a number of disease states, i.e. heart failure, constrictive pericarditis and left-to-right shunts, there is no rise in blood pressure in Phase II nor any further rise in blood pressure and slowing of the heart rate in Phase IV. Even in extensive pulmonary disease, however, there are normal responses in all four phases.

165 Potassium ferricyanide stains Prussian blue in the presence of Fe^{2+}; the diagnosis is haemochromatosis. In its idiopathic form, this is an autosomal recessively inherited disorder of iron storage. A number of internal organs (such as the liver, spleen, pancreas and bone marrow) are saturated with iron, probably due to an excessive uptake of iron by abnormally functioning enterocytes in the gut. The heart also takes up an excess of iron, to a greater extent than does skeletal muscle. Melanin is deposited in the skin, hence the term 'bronzed diabetes'. The severity of disease from the cardiovascular point of view depends upon the degree of myocardial infiltration with iron. Initially, the perinuclear region of the myocardial fibre is involved, then the whole fibre. Degeneration and fibrosis follow, ultimately leading to a dilated cardiomyopathy, sometimes via a restrictive phase. Atypical chest pain and (usually atrial) arrhythmias are common. Treatment is by the management of arrhythmias and symptoms of cardiac failure, as well as with more specific measures for the iron overload. These would include repeated venesection and the use of chelating agents, such as desferrioxamine. In view of the genetic nature of the disease, screening of siblings should be considered. (However, even siblings are unlikely to be affected because the disorder is recessively inherited, so two heterozygous parents are required.)

166 i. The ECG shows atrial premature beats (APBs). APBs characteristically have an abnormally shaped P wave (the P′ wave) prior to the next expected QRS complex. The PR interval is usually similar to (or a little longer than) the standard PR interval. Depending upon the site of origin of the APB, the characteristics of the atrioventricular node and the presence or absence of any accessory pathways, the APB may be normally conducted, aberrantly conducted, or completely blocked.
ii. There are many causes of APBs, including structural heart disease (coronary artery disease, angina, acute myocardial infarction, cardiomyopathy, heart failure, myocarditis and mitral valve prolapse), thyrotoxicosis, anxiety and high catecholamine drive, caffeine, alcohol, volatile anaesthetics, digoxin, hypokalaemia, hypomagnesaemia, pneumonia and bronchial carcinoma. Treatment is directed at the alleviation of provoking factors. Specific treatment is only indicated for the relief of symptoms, since the prognosis is excellent. Of the available drugs, beta-blockers are probably the most effective.

167 A 50-year-old South American man was admitted to a London hospital with worsening breathlessness, but no history of chest pain. He was not diabetic. On close questioning, he admitted to having been acutely ill with breathlessness and fever, necessitating hospital admission, 10 years previously, when in Buenos Aires.
i. What do you see?
ii. Suggest a diagnosis.

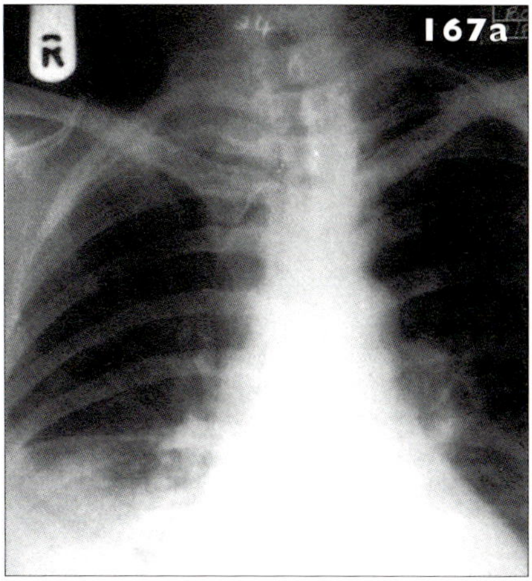
167a

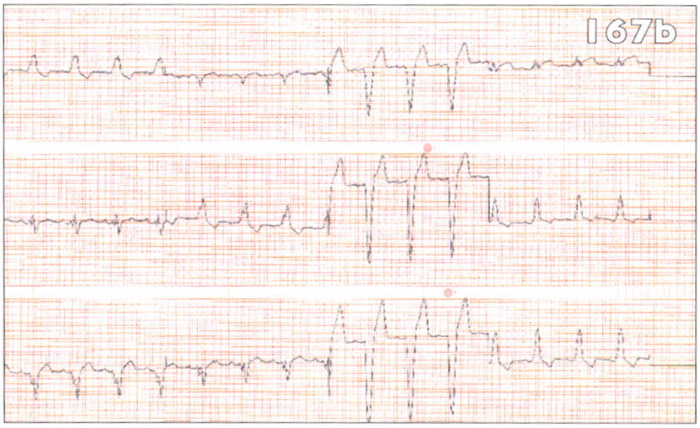
167b

168 This patient, who was in atrial fibrillation and had a pan-systolic murmur audible at the apex radiating to the axilla, was receiving long-term follow-up after rheumatic fever 28 years previously. He was a little breathless in the course of his work as a university lecturer in classics. His thoughts had returned again to cardiac surgery, an option mentioned some years before.

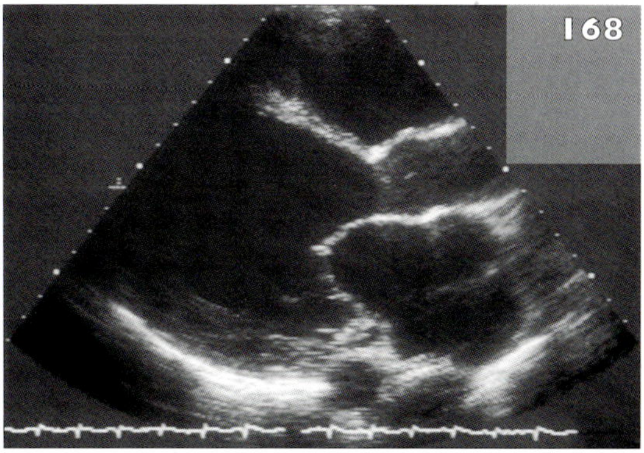
168

i. What does this investigation show?
ii. Does it help to decide when (if at all) to refer this patient for surgery?
iii. What degree of functional improvement do you expect?

167 **i.** The chest radiograph (**167a**) shows cardiomegaly and the ECG (**167b**) shows left bundle branch block and left axis deviation.
ii. This man's illness began with the acute febrile illness in Argentina. He had Chagas' disease (trypanosomiasis), a common South American cause of chronic heart disease. Transmission to man of *Trypanosoma cruzii* in the faeces of the insect vector during blood feeding produces an acute systemic illness and infective myocarditis, with acute dilatation of the heart, heart failure and electrocardiographic abnormalities. After the acute illness, a chronic phase follows, characterised by myocardial scarring which typically involves the conducting tissues. Although not shown in this example, the atrioventricular node is also often involved, leading to atrioventricular block; globally, Chagas' disease is probably the leading cause of the latter. Lesions of the cardiac nerves are also common, with alteration of the normal regulation of heart rate period. In common with this, the intramuscular ganglia of hollow viscera are also affected. A probable mechanism underlying myoneuronal involvement is an autoimmune cross-reaction between antigens exposed on *Trypanosoma cruzii* and those of the host neural tissues.

168 **i.** The investigation is a 2D echocardiogram. It shows thickening of the mitral valve and reduced movement of the cusps. The left atrium is dilated, as is the left ventricle. In conjunction with the clinical history, it is clear that this patient has dominant mitral regurgitation of rheumatic origin.
ii. The functional status of this patient is severely impaired. His occupation is a sedentary one and, despite that, he is still becoming breathless (i.e. probably Grade III dyspnoea according to the New York Heart Association classification). The left ventricular dilatation suggests that left ventricular function is already significantly impaired. Symptoms (which occur late in mitral regurgitation) and/or a left ventricular end diastolic dimension >7.0 cm or a systolic dimension >4.5 cm are indications for mitral valve replacement. Thus, this patient is long overdue for surgery. He should have received regular follow-up to document the development of symptoms and – most importantly – for serial measurements of the left ventricular end systolic and end diastolic dimensions and for the derivation of left ventricular ejection fraction.
iii. Complete restoration of left ventricular function will not occur, since the left ventricle is already damaged. Further deterioration may not be prevented by surgery at this late stage. Preservation of the tensing apparatus – papillary muscle and chordae – and of annular continuity by mitral valve repair rather than replacement best preserves left ventricular function, but is often not possible in rheumatic mitral valve disease. On the medical front, an angiotensin-converting enzyme (ACE) inhibitor should be prescribed and continued post-operatively.

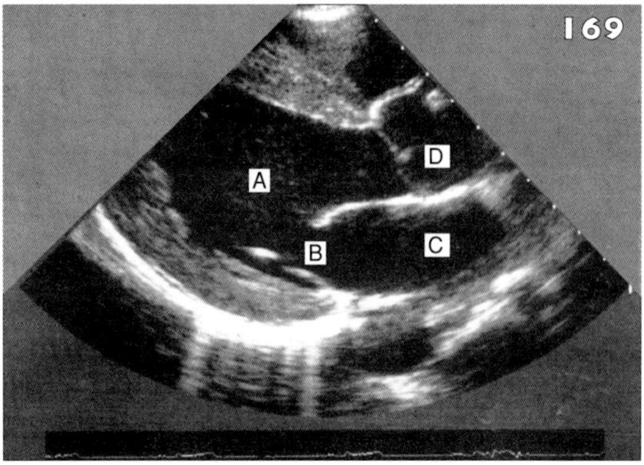

169 A 27-year-old women was 20 weeks pregnant. A soft ejection systolic murmur had been heard at the antenatal clinic. Her pulse was 73 b.p.m., blood pressure 105/55 mmHg, and she was asymptomatic. The investigation shown was performed. (*NB* Doppler studies were normal.)

i. What are the structures A–D?

ii. What abnormalities do you see?

iii. What is the most likely cause of this woman's murmur?

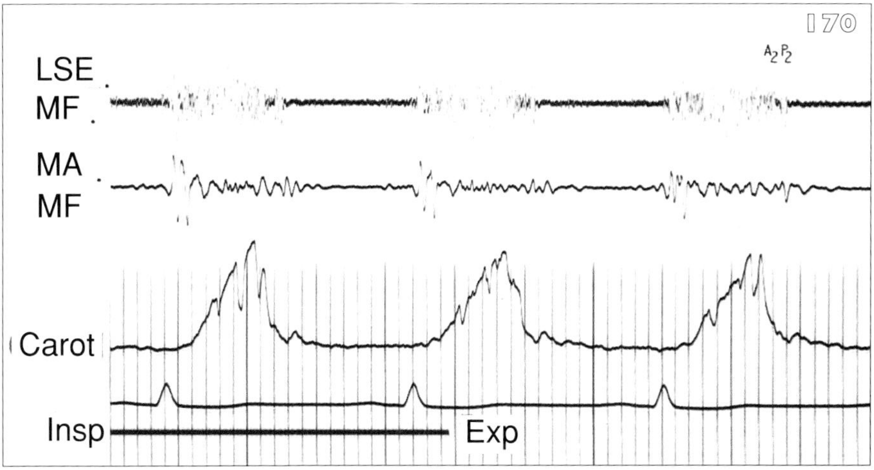

170 These sound traces (medium frequency filtered, obtained from the left sternal edge and left axilla) and indirect carotid artery pressure traces were obtained from a patient with documented exercise-provoked syncope. (LSE, left sternal edge; MF, medium frequency filtered; MA, mitral area; Carot, carotid; Insp, inspiratory phase; Exp, expiratory phase.)

i. What is the cause of the patient's syncope?

ii. What would you do about it?

169 i. A 2D echocardiogram, parasternal long-axis view, is shown. The structures labelled are: A, left ventricular cavity; B, mitral valve; C, left atrium; and D, aortic valve.
ii. The echocardiogram is normal.
iii. Clinically, this young woman is well and asymptomatic, with appropriate heart rate and blood pressure. The murmur is most likely due to an increased flow of blood because of the increased stroke volume in pregnancy. During pregnancy, the blood volume increases by 20–100% (mean 50%) from the resting value, with the steepest rate of increase occurring in mid-pregnancy. This may be due, at least in part, to an oestrogen-provoked increase in renin, promoting aldosterone secretion and sodium and water retention. (The increase in plasma volume is greater than the increase in red cell mass – the physiological anaemia of pregnancy.) In addition to the increase in stroke volume which commences from the first trimester, there is also an increase in resting heart rate of 10–20 b.p.m. in the third trimester. Peripheral resistance falls, partly due to the fetoplacental unit having a low resistance circulation. The blood pressure falls accordingly, being minimal in the second trimester. At echocardiography, a measure of volume loading of both ventricles is typical of pregnancy, although the chamber dimensions differ very little from the non-pregnant state.

170 i. The phonocardiogram shows the murmur of (severe) aortic stenosis. There is no ejection click because the valve is calcified. In aortic stenosis, left ventricular ejection is prolonged and the aortic component of the second heart sound is delayed and soft. It can occur at the same time as the pulmonary component, producing a single second sound during inspiration, when the pulmonary component of the second sound occurs later. This paradoxical splitting of the second heart sound (pulmonary and aortic components of the second heart sound moving closer together during inspiration) can be seen in the traces. However, neither a fourth nor a third heart sound can be seen on the trace. The carotid trace shows a typical slow-rising pressure wave with systolic vibrations on the upstroke.
ii. For both prognostic and symptomatic reasons, the patient should have an aortic valve replacement. The operation is usually extremely successful, with age being no bar to surgery. There is no case for medical management, other than in mild-to-moderate asymptomatic cases. Despite initial promise, balloon valvoplasty has not been shown to improve outlook in patients with valvar calcification.

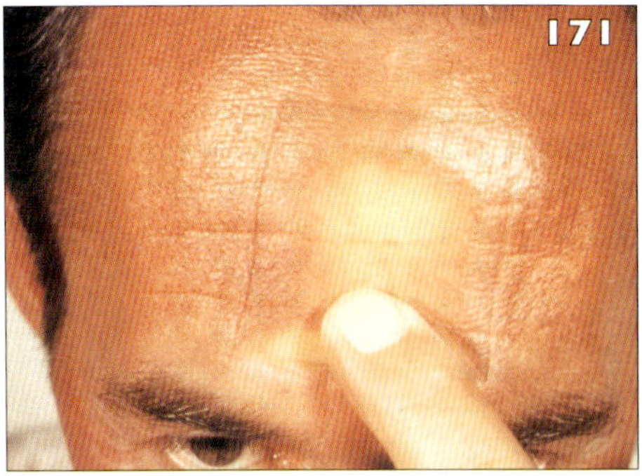

171 A 56-year-old man complained of flushing. He also noticed a feeling of fullness in the chest, neck and face, especially on bending down. On examination in the hospital out-patient department, the physician noticed the physical sign shown.
i. What physical sign is shown and what is the underlying diagnosis?
ii. What typical physical signs would you expect to find?

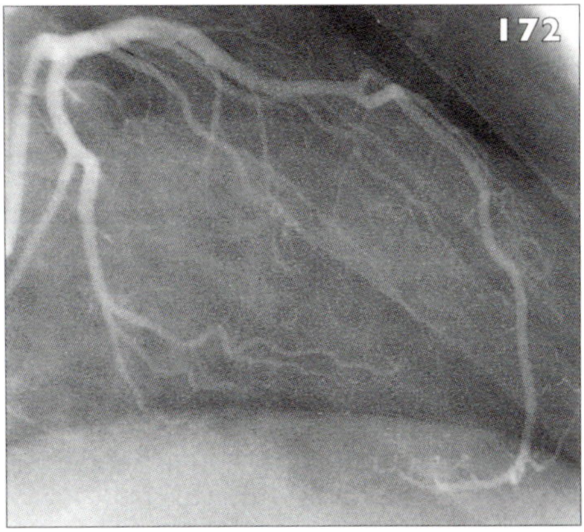

172 This is a coronary arteriogram.
i. Which artery is this?
ii. List the branches of this vessel.

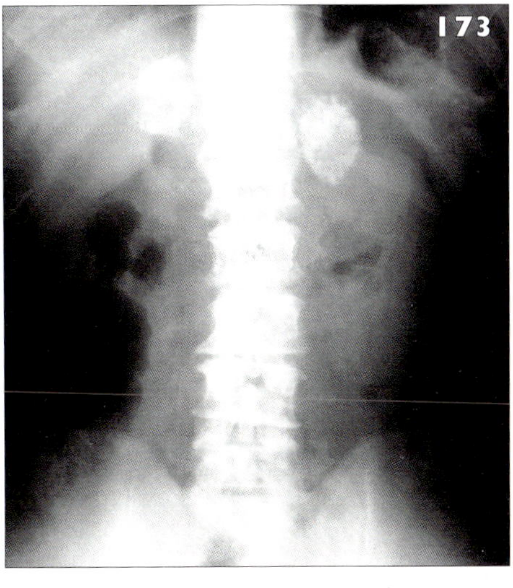

173 A 40-year-old man who lived alone and who did irregular labouring work felt vaguely weaker and weaker over a period of 3 months. On one occasion he collapsed and was brought to the emergency room. He was found to have a pulse of 74 b.p.m. and blood pressure of 90/50 mmHg lying and 75/45 mmHg standing. The initial blood investigations revealed sodium, 132 mmol/l, potassium, 5.3 mmol/l and urea of 6.0 mmol/l (BUN, 14.8 mg/dl). Why was this man hypotensive?

171 **i.** A carcinoid flush is shown; the underlying diagnosis is carcinoid syndrome.
ii. The carcinoid syndrome is due to the excessive secretion of 5-hydroxytryptamine (5-HT) and vasoactive peptides by neoplastic enterochromaffin cells. Typically, the primary tumour is located in the gut and rarely in the ovary or lung. In the last case, release of the 5-HT and peptides into the systemic circulation can occur from the primary tumour. In the more common gut location of the tumours, metastasis to the liver with release of 5-HT and peptides into the hepatic veins occurs before presentation. There is cardiac involvement in about half the cases of carcinoid, usually in the form of grey fibrous tissue plaques on the endovascular aspect of the right heart, vena cava and coronary sinus. Mixed tricuspid and pulmonary valve disease is common and often ultimately fatal. In the rare cases of lung carcinoid, left-sided heart lesions can be found. Besides the signs of tricuspid and/or pulmonary valve disease, other physical signs common in carcinoid syndrome are cutaneous flushing, telangiectasia of the face and bronchoconstriction.

172 **i.** This is the left coronary artery.
ii. The left coronary artery commences as the left main stem and divides into the left anterior descending artery and the circumflex artery. In some patients it gives off a third branch between the anterior descending and circumflex branches, known as the intermediate artery. The left anterior descending artery has one or two main diagonal arteries which supply the anterior aspect of the left ventricle. It also provides several smaller diagonal and septal branches. The anterosuperior aspect of the ventricular septum is supplied by the left coronary artery. The circumflex artery also has one or two large marginal branches, which supply the posterior aspect of the left ventricle, as do a number of smaller posterior ventricular branches. In about one-fifth of the population, the posterior descending artery and the artery to the atrioventricular node arise from the circumflex artery. Such patients are said to have a dominant left coronary system.

173 This man has obvious postural hypotension. Causes of this are primary or secondary hypoadrenalism, autonomic neuropathy and dehydration due to diuretics. The electrolyte data indicate primary hypoadrenalism. The ultimate cause, i.e. tuberculous (rather than autoimmune) adrenalitis can be determined from the abdominal radiograph; there is calcification of the suprarenal glands. Further investigations would show reduced serum aldosterone, high plasma renin and (possibly) low blood glucose . Adrenal antibodies may be detectable (in cases due to autoimmune adrenalitis). Plasma cortisol is low; several estimates may be necessary. The short corticotrophin stimulation test will demonstrate an impaired cortisol response. The chest radiograph may also show signs of tuberculosis. Treatment includes, in the acute situation, resuscitation with intravenous fluids (repeated to achieve haemodynamic stability and guided by central venous pressure monitoring), and administration of intravenous hydrocortisone and intravenous dextrose for hypoglycaemia. In the longer term, tuberculosis must be treated if present; mineralocorticoid replacement may require regular fludrocortisone.

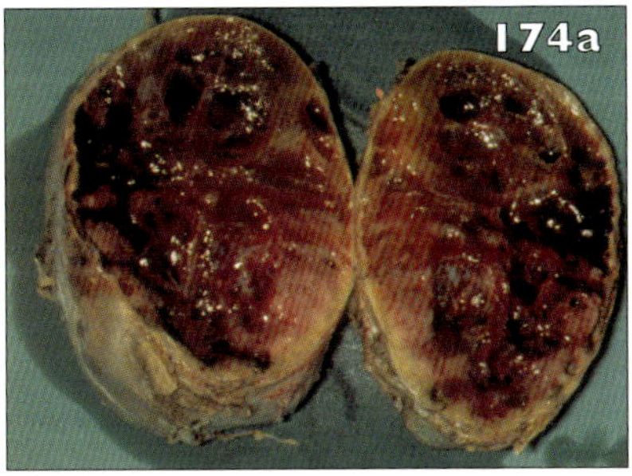
174a

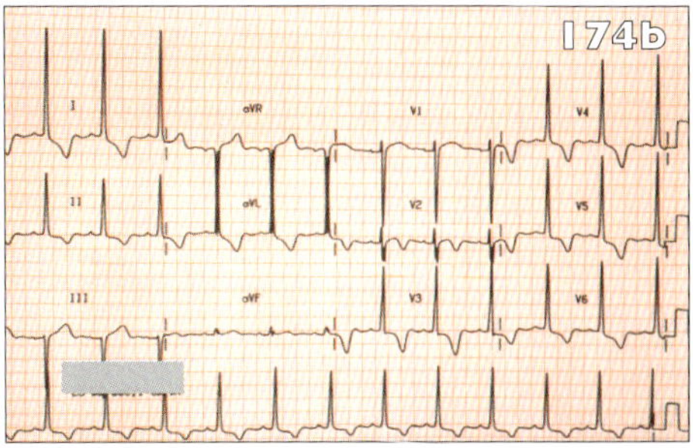
174b

174 This 32-year-old woman complained of headaches, sweating, and palpitations for 2 years. She had been noted to have hypertension, but had not been investigated. A diagnosis was eventually made following which she had surgical treatment. A pathological specimen (**174a**) and an ECG (**174b**) are shown.

i. What is shown in **174a**?

ii. What is the ECG finding in **174b**?

175 A 68-year-old woman, successfully treated a few weeks previously for dizzy spells, started to feel giddy once again. She was referred back to her cardiologist who had an ECG performed.

i. How had she been treated?

ii. What problem has developed?

iii. What treatment options are available?

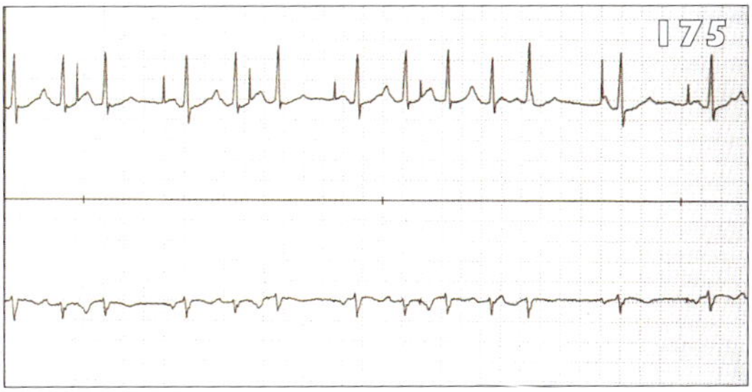
175

176 The ECG shown was obtained from a 55-year-old patient who attended his family practitioner after an acute episode of chest pain.

i. What is the diagnosis?

ii. What is the likely site of the lesion responsible for this?

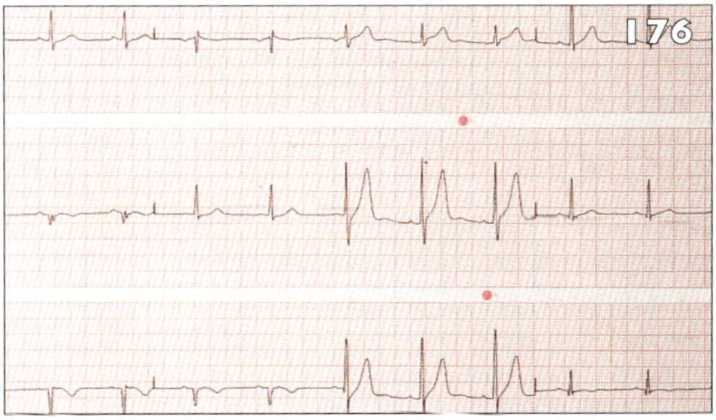
176

174 **i.** **174a** shows a macroscopic specimen of a phaeochromocytoma.
ii. **174b** shows an ECG with the voltage criteria of left ventricular hypertrophy. The patient had secondary hypertension from a phaeochromocytoma, which led to left ventricular hypertrophy.

Phaeochromocytoma is a catecholamine-secreting tumour of chromaffin cells, of which 90% are found in the adrenal medulla. Extra-adrenal sites include the sympathetic trunk, in which case the cervical site has the highest preponderance, paragangliomas within the abdomen, and tumours in the bladder. Most tumours are benign, 10% are malignant and 10% are bilateral. Most cases are sporadic, but familial forms are recognised and often form part of a syndrome, such as multiple endocrine neoplasia (Type 2), von Hippel–Lindau syndrome and neurofibromatosis. The incidence of the tumour among patients with hypertension is 0.1%. The most common symptoms are headache, sweating and palpitations. Hypertension is usually sustained and postural hypotension occurs in 70% of cases. Investigation and treatment are discussed in **221**. Left ventricular hypertrophy on the ECG is diagnosed when the sum of the R wave in V5 or V6 and the S wave in V1 exceeds 35 mm. ST segment depression and T wave inversion in the leads facing the left ventricle are occasionally present. Echocardiography is much superior to the ECG in the diagnosis of left ventricular hypertrophy.

175 **i.** This woman had sinoatrial disease which caused symptomatic bradycardiac episodes for which she was treated by insertion of a permanent ventricular pacing system (VVI mode).
ii. The trace shows a number of natural beats with a paced beat occurring inappropriately soon after the natural beat; there is certainly no long pause before the paced beat comes in (see arrow on trace). The pacing system is failing to sense and to be inhibited by the patient's intrinsic beats. The reason for the failure to sense may be that the intrinsic R wave is too small, there may be too low a slew rate (rate of rise of endocardial potential: dV/dt), or the pacing unit may be too insensitive.
iii. In this clinical situation, reprogramming of the system to increase the R wave sensitivity might be of benefit. However it is likely that the pacemaker lead will need to be repositioned, or possibly replaced with a new lead with a porous tip electrode.

176 **i.** The ECG shows Q waves in II, III, and aVF, as well as tall R waves in leads V1–V3. The T waves in the latter leads are also tall and symmetrical. The diagnosis is an inferior infarct with extensive posterior extension. In true posterior infarction, the posterior wall electrical contribution is lost and septal activation is followed by activation of the free (anterior) wall of the right ventricle. Both forces are now positively oriented towards electrodes at V1 and V2, producing tall R waves in these leads.
Similarly, since the T wave vector is usually directed away from infarcted myocardium, the T waves 'viewed' from the rightward anterior chest leads (V1 and V2) will be positive and tall.
ii. An occlusion of the right coronary artery is most likely, since in 85% of people the

177 A 27-year-old man, who had recently immigrated, was reviewed in the cardiology out-patient department because of an asymptomatic murmur. On examination, a systolic thrill could be felt to the left of the manubriosternal joint and, on auscultation, a click and loud systolic murmur was heard.
i. Can you see any abnormality on this patient's chest radiograph?
ii. What is the diagnosis?
iii. How would you investigate and manage this patient?

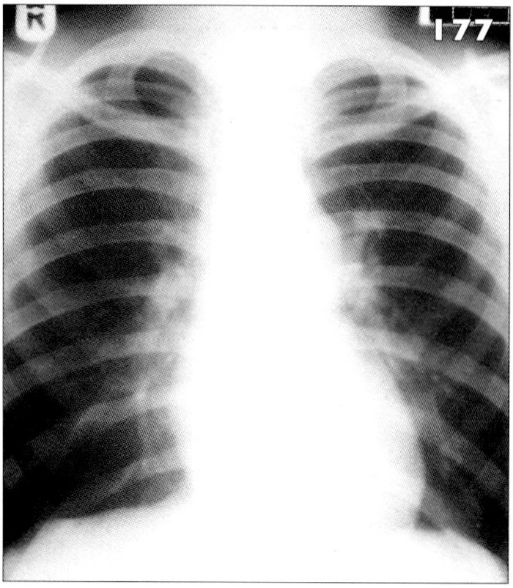

178 A 37-year-old woman presented with chest tightness and palpitations. Subsequently, she complained of muscular weakness, nausea, dizziness, and headaches. Her blood pressure was 180/110 mmHg and her electrolytes are as follows: sodium, 144 mmol/l; potassium, 3.3 mmol/l; urea, 8 mmol/l (BUN, 22.4 mg/dl); glucose, 5 mmol/l (90 mg/dl); bicarbonate, 30 mmol/l. A further investigation is shown.
i. Suggest a diagnosis.
ii. What is the investigation shown?

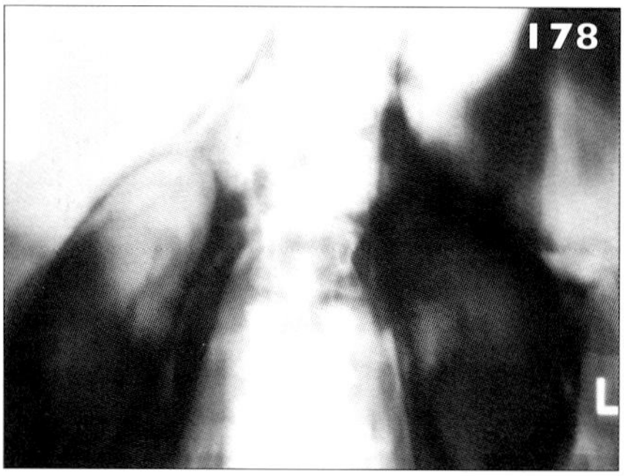

179 These are separate rhythm strips from a 24-hour ECG study on a 70-year-old man with chest pain accompanied by dizziness.
i. List two abnormalities visible when the patient experiences chest pain.
ii. Which single test would you request to aid his management?

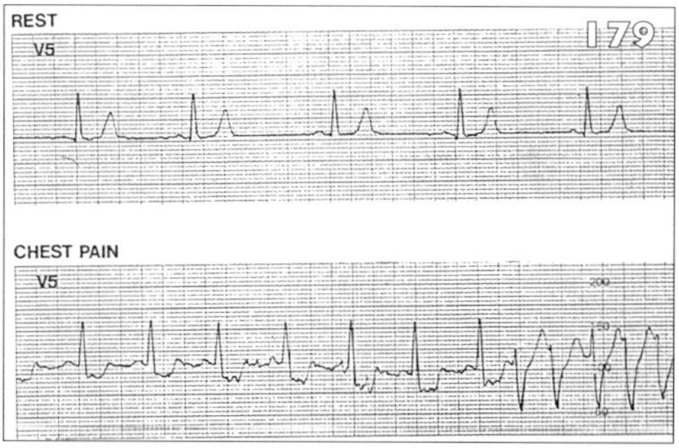

177 i. The chest radiograph shows post-stenotic dilatation of the pulmonary artery.
ii. In the context of the classic auscultatory findings (systolic click and murmur best heard in area of the pulmonary valve), the diagnosis is pulmonary stenosis.
iii. The increased right ventricular afterload due to stenosis of the pulmonary valve has the predictable effect of provoking right ventricular hypertrophy. Reflecting this, the right ventricular ECG will typically show right axis deviation, right atrial enlargement and right ventricular hypertrophy. Echocardiography can identify any associated lesions, such as atrial septal defect, ventricular septal defect, or patent ductus arteriosus. Cardiac catheterisation is of no additional use. Percutaneous balloon valvoplasty can be performed (see **112**). If there is more complicated anatomical derangement, surgical valvotomy and repair of the associated lesions should be performed.

178 i. This young woman with significant hypertension and the range of other symptoms listed had Conn's syndrome. This disorder is caused by an aldosterone-secreting adenoma or hyperplasia of the adrenal cortex. The principal action of aldosterone is the promotion of sodium reabsorption in exchange for potassium and hydrogen at the distal nephron. It is a rare disorder – <0.1% of cases of hypertension. The electrolyte data presented give the clue to the diagnosis, as there is a raised sodium, low potassium and raised bicarbonate (metabolic alkalosis).
ii. The figure is a tomogram of the abdomen, showing an adrenal macroadenoma. Iodocholesterol scanning is valuable, especially after a dexamethasone suppression test. (The latter test confirms that the high levels of circulating aldosterone cannot be lowered by manipulation of the intrinsic feedback mechanisms). The adrenal cortical adenoma selectively takes up the tracer. CT scanning of the adrenals can enable more detailed localisation.
iii. Treatment with spironolactone is indicated if the cause is adrenal hyperplasia. If an adenoma has been identified as the cause of the Conn's syndrome, then surgical excision should be performed.

179 i. There is significant ST segment depression followed by a run of ventricular tachycardia.
ii. The most common cause of ventricular tachycardia is myocardial ischaemia. He is likely to have important coronary artery disease and it is therefore essential to perform coronary angiography. The other possibility in this case is severe aortic stenosis – if there is any evidence of this on clinical examination, echocardiography should be requested. Aortic stenosis can also be diagnosed during left heart catheterisation at the time of coronary angiography; however, it is not always wise to try to cross the aortic valve when it is heavily calcified, so it is preferable to assess the severity of aortic stenosis by Doppler studies during echocardiography. (Other causes of ventricular tachycardia are discussed in **214**.)

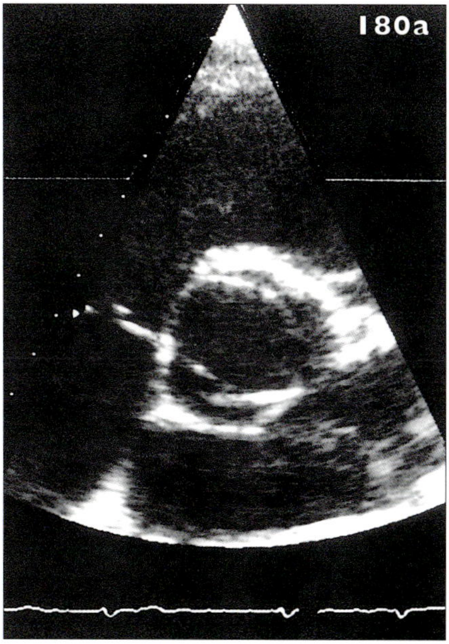

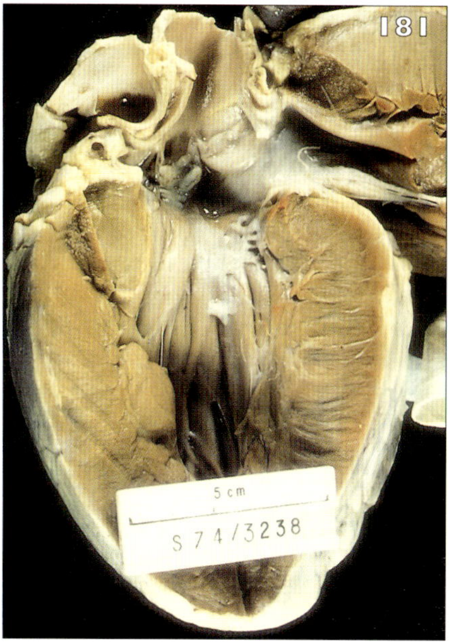

180 A 25-year-old man followed annually for a 'murmur' had the echocardiographic appearance shown in **182a**.
i. What is the abnormality shown?
ii. How common is it?
iii. What is the natural history?

181 A 40-year-old man collapsed suddenly and died when gardening. At post-mortem the appearance of his heart was as shown.
i. What is the diagnosis?
ii. What are the chances that his son will develop the same condition?

182 What is this investigation and what does it show?

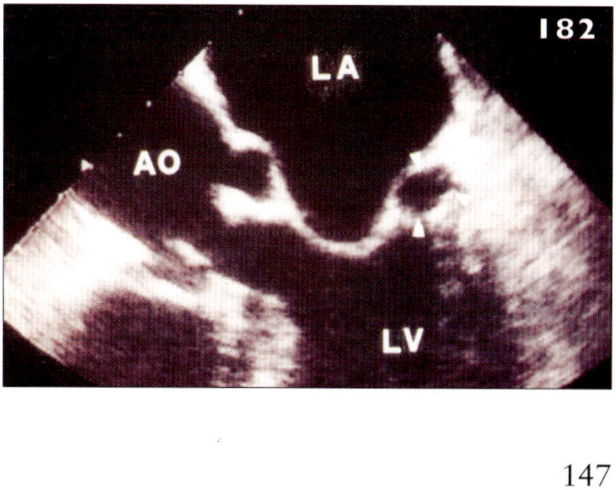

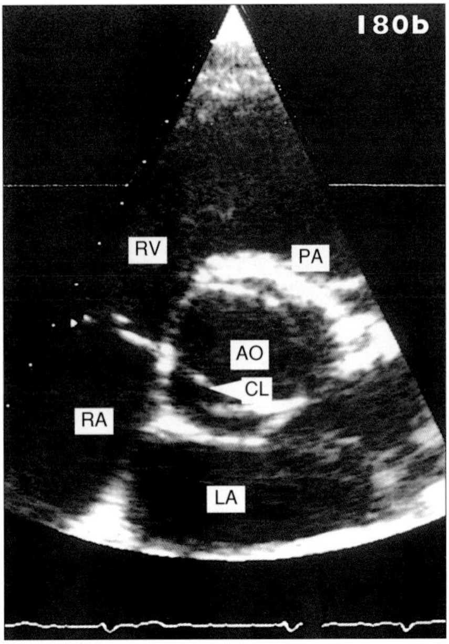

180 **i.** As shown and labelled in **180b**, the parasternal short axis 2D echocardiographic view of the aortic valve (AO, in the middle of the field of view) does not show the usual three valve leaflets (clockwise from the top of this view, these would be the right coronary leaflet, the left coronary leaflet, and the non-coronary leaflet). This aortic valve is bicuspid; there is only one closure line between the leaflets. The valve is not calcified. (RA, right atrium; RV, right ventricle; LA, left atrium; AO, aortic valve; PA, pulmonary artery; CL, closure line.)
ii. The incidence of the abnormality is 1–2% of the general population, with the disorder being more prevalent among males.
iii. Generally, about one-third of patients with bicuspid aortic valve develop significant aortic stenosis later in life, when the valve calcifies; however, between one-third and a half of all subjects with a bicuspid aortic valve remain asymptomatic.

181 **i.** This post-mortem heart shows gross hypertrophy of all the myocardial walls, especially the ventricular septum. The diagnosis is hypertrophic cardiomyopathy.
ii. An autosomal dominant mode of inheritance for hypertrophic cardiomyopathy was suggested originally by Teare, so there would be a 50% chance of the son inheriting the mutant gene. Approximately 60% of cases are familial. The others arise by spontaneous mutation. Genetic defects have been identified in the β-myosin heavy chain, tropomyosin and troponin C genes.

182 This is a transoesophageal echocardiogram and it shows the left atrium, left ventricle and aorta; there is a mitral paravalvar abscess. Transoesophageal echocardiography has been of immense value in both the diagnosis and monitoring of treatment of endocarditis, since it allows an unobstructed near view of the valves and yields images of very high quality. Abscess formation in endocarditis is particularly common in staphylococcal endocarditis. The site of suppuration is commonly the base of the valve and the valve annulus. Aortic valve abscesses can (and frequently do) extend into the surrounding structures leading to, e.g., interruption of atrioventricular conduction (when the bundle branches are affected). Impaired myocardial contraction due to myocardial abscess formation, fistula formation, and, rarely, aneurysm formation on the valve or annulus, or to rupture of the chordae tendineae or papillary muscles may occur.

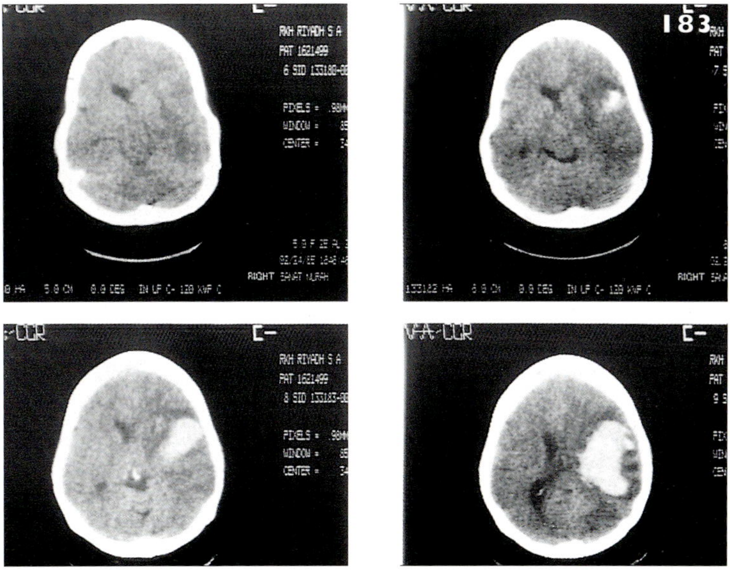

183 A 27-year-old male drug abuser was admitted after a month of worsening breathlessness and malaise. On examination, he was pyrexial (temperature 38°C), tachycardic (128 b.p.m.), and with a blood pressure of 105/50 mmHg. Mid-systolic and early diastolic murmurs were noted, as well as basal crackles on auscultation of the chest. After 3 weeks of intravenous antibiotics, his condition had improved considerably. However, one morning he was found on the floor of his room, having a seizure. After the immediate management, the appearances shown were obtained.

i. What is the investigation and what does it show?

ii. Give two mechanisms whereby this complication may develop.

184 A 55-year-old man was admitted with severe central chest pain at rest, which was not relieved by sublingual nitrates.

i. What are the abnormalities on this ECG?

ii. What is the probable diagnosis?

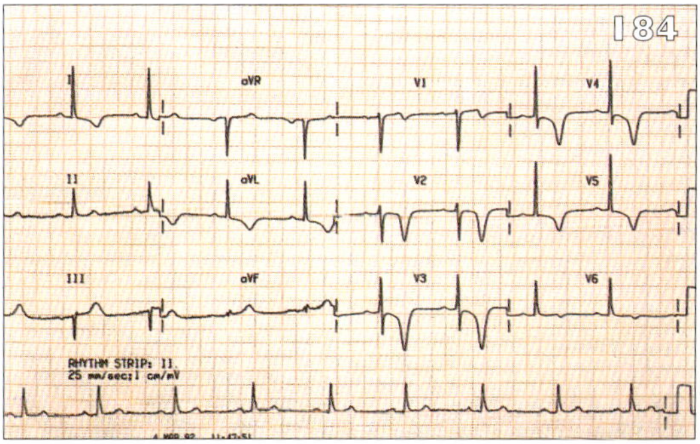

183 i. Shown are CT scans of the brain. They show a haemorrhagic mass in the right temporal lobe due to a ruptured mycotic aneurysm.
ii. Mycotic aneurysms are found in 10–15% of autopsy cases of patients with infective endocarditis. They are probably caused by blood-borne bacteria-containing emboli entering the vessel wall via the vasa vasorum or from the vascular lumen at points of endothelial injury. Lesions are more common at branch points of the vascular system. Although many mycotic aneurysms are not detected clinically, causing no symptoms, they do occasionally rupture – intracerebral sites are the most dangerous for this and account for about half of the mycotic aneurysms detected clinically. More generally, cerebral symptoms may be the presenting feature in about 20% of cases of endocarditis, with either non-specific symptoms, meningitis, encephalitis, single or multiple cerebral abscesses and embolic infarction, besides the mycotic aneurysm formation described here.

184 i. There is ST depression and deep T wave inversion in leads I, aVl, and V2–V5. There are no Q waves and there is no loss of R waves.
ii. The history is suggestive of myocardial infarction. The ECG changes probably represent a subendocardial anterolateral myocardial infarction, but this can only be confirmed by serial ECGs to demonstrate persistence of the ECG changes despite intravenous nitrates, whereas if the changes were due to ischaemia they would resolve. Cardiac enzymes would also be modestly elevated in the case of infarction.

Subendocardial (or non-Q wave myocardial infarction) is usually due to subacute coronary artery occlusion. The hospital mortality is only 2% as compared with full thickness or Q wave infarction, where the mortality is 10–12%. These patients often proceed to develop Q wave infarction within a year and therefore the 1-year mortality is much higher. For this reason it is appropriate to investigate these patients with coronary angiography and ambulatory 24-hour ECG monitoring as there is a higher incidence of arrhythmias. Treatment is with intravenous heparin and nitrates. Thrombolysis has not been shown to reduce early mortality.

185 This patient complained of dizziness on exertion. What is the ECG diagnosis?

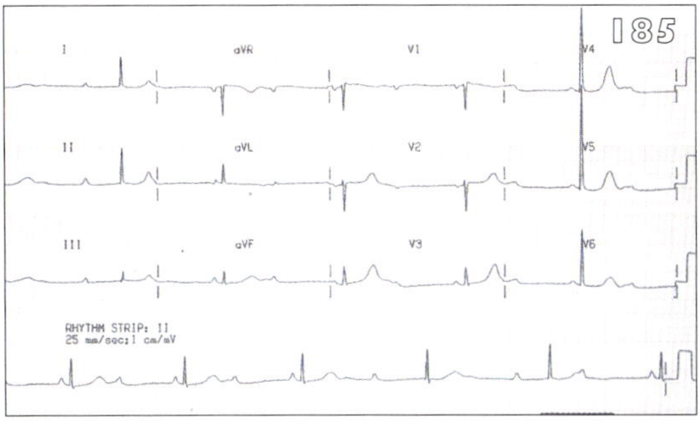

186 The tracing shown was obtained in the pre-surgical investigations performed on a 58-year-old woman. (PA, pulmonary area; HF, high frequency filter; MA, mitral area; BA, brachial artery; LV, left vetricle; LA, left atrium; SM, systolic murmur; DM, diastolic murmur.)
What is the diagnosis?

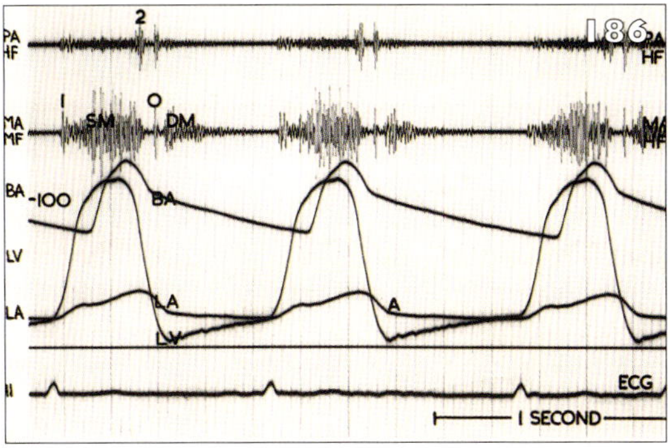

187 This exercise test was performed on a 46-year-old man with central chest pain on exertion. He was a smoker and had a family history of ischaemic heart disease. His physical examination was normal, but the test was terminated due to chest pain.
i. How would you interpret the test?
ii. What is the likelihood of his having coronary artery disease?

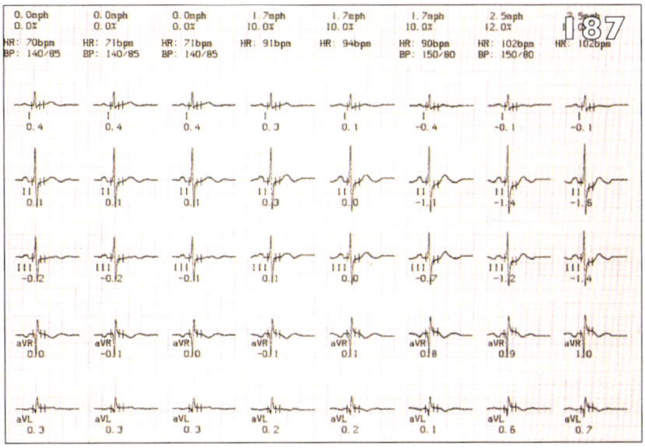

185 There is evidence of Mobitz Type II atrioventricular block with 2:1 atrioventricular conduction. The atrial rate is 100 b.p.m. and the ventricular rate is 50 b.p.m. Mobitz Type II block is due to impaired conduction in the bundle of His or bundle branches. This type of bradyarrhythmia is likely to progress to third degree atrioventricular block and sudden death, so it is an indication for permanent pacemaker implantation.

186 The tracing shows that at the end of isovolumic relaxation and opening of the mitral valve, the left ventricular pressure falls below that of the left atrium, i.e. there is a gradient between the left atrium and left ventricle during diastole. Thus, the patient has mitral stenosis. The simultaneous phonocardiogram shows a loud first heart sound, coincident with the abrupt closure of the mitral valve leaflets which come together during the rapid rise in left ventricular pressure, the leaflets having remained apart later into diastole than normal. There is a systolic murmur due to moderate accompanying mitral regurgitation. The second heart sound can be seen, followed by an opening snap (O). The large pressure gradient between the left atrium and left ventricle causes a sudden tensing of the mitral valve ring to accompany the opening of the mitral leaflets, which bow towards the left ventricle because of commissural fusion. After the opening snap, there is a mid-diastolic murmur (DM) during trans-mitral flow through the stenosed valve. In mild cases, the diastolic murmur is quite short and the left ventricular and left atrial pressures equalise prior to the first heart sound. In severe cases, when the pressures fail to equalise throughout diastole, the diastolic murmur continues up to the next first heart sound. The patient is in atrial fibrillation (note the absence of P waves on the ECG) and there is no pre-systolic murmur.

187 **i.** Two stages of the Bruce protocol exercise test were completed. The heart rate went up from 70 to 102 b.p.m. ST segment depression developed in leads II, III and aVf and reached a maximum of 1.5 mm. The test is positive at a low workload.
ii. There is a high chance of the patient having coronary artery disease. A test is interpreted as positive if there is planar ST segment depression of 1.5 mm in one or more leads. When chest pain occurs in association with ST segment depression, the sensitivity of the test increases. Chest pain of angina quality induced by exercise in the absence of ECG changes should be taken seriously, because ischaemia in the posterior ventricular wall is not always demonstrated by the ECG. The high probability of important coronary artery disease is suggested by ST segment depression occurring at a heart rate below 120 b.p.m. (in the absence of beta-blockers), a failure of the blood pressure to rise or drop by 10 mmHg, ventricular arrhythmias developing at a low workload and a poor exercise tolerance.

Contraindications to exercise testing are severe symptomatic left ventricular outflow tract obstruction, myocarditis, pericarditis, left ventricular failure, complete heart block, unstable angina, ventricular arrhythmias, renal failure, febrile illness and dissecting aortic aneurysm. (Causes of false positive tests are discussed in **79**.)

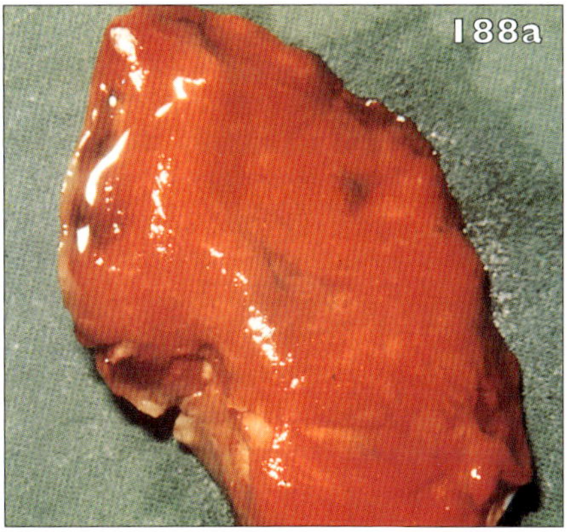

188a

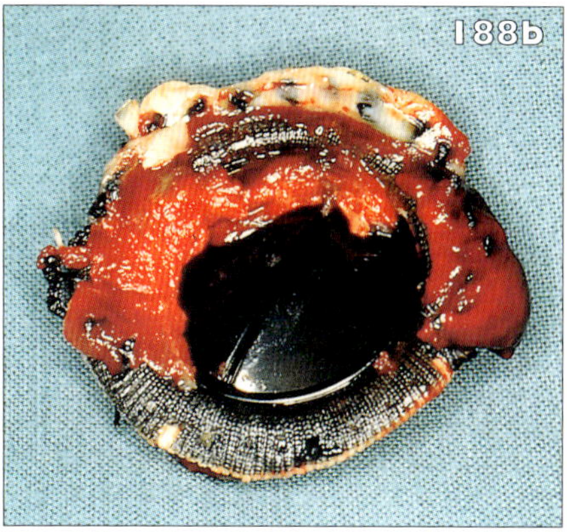

188b

188 A 50-year-old alcoholic patient underwent open-heart surgery for a long-standing 'problem with his breathing'. After 3 years, when his drink problem had become quite severe, the man collapsed a couple of times, underwent investigation and had a further operation. What do you think happened?

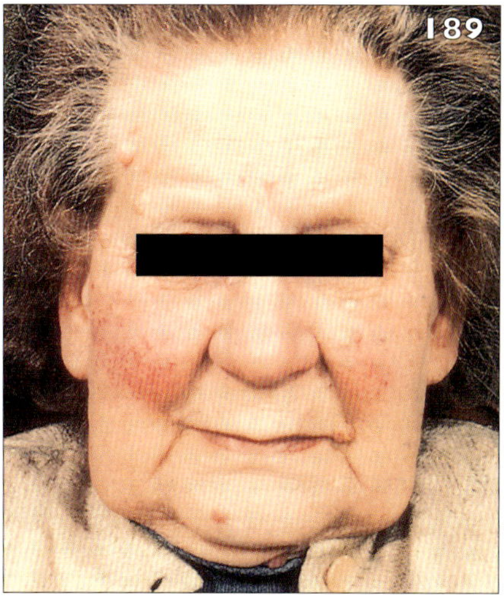

189

189 This 70-year-old woman was referred to the cardiology out-patient clinic after complaining of chest pain on exertion. What are your initial thoughts?

190 A 14-year-old boy was treated for an acute leukaemia. After his third course of treatment he developed breathlessness on mild exertion. On examination he had the signs of biventricular failure and his haemoglobin was 10 g/dl. What is the most likely explanation for this?

188 **188a** shows a large clot removed surgically from the left atrium and **188b** a stenosed St Jude mechanical valve prosthesis. The clinical case history was as follows. The patient had rheumatic fever at the age of 16 years. Subsequently, he developed mitral stenosis which caused breathlessness on exertion. After several years, the problem became more severe until he underwent mitral valve replacement with a St Jude prosthesis. (The latter is a bileaflet valve, with two semicircular occluding leaflets made of pyrolytic carbon. There is generally a lower risk of leaflet entrapment than in the single tilting disc prostheses, such as the Bjork Shiley valve, but as with all mechanical valves, indefinite anticoagulation is mandatory.) As the patient's personal problems worsened, he resorted increasingly to alcohol and his drug compliance declined until he stopped taking anticoagulants. The episodes of collapse were due to the atrial clot acting as a ball valve. The only treatment for the condition is replacement of the stenosed valve prosthesis. Thrombolytic therapy may be tried if the thrombosis has occurred fairly acutely. There is some risk of causing embolism, but this is a lesser risk than that of repeat surgery.

189 This woman, who subsequently gave a classic description of angina of effort, has a hypothyroid facies. A low plasma thyroxine and raised thyroid-stimulating hormone levels were found at laboratory investigation. Cardiological features of hypothyroidism include, on examination, bradycardia and sometimes signs of heart failure. Hypotension may be evident and the heart sounds may be quiet. On further investigation of the patient, the chest radiograph showed cardiomegaly due (chiefly) to a pericardial effusion, confirmed by subsequent echocardiography. The resting ECG showed sinus bradycardia with prolongation of the QT interval. Overall, the QRS complexes were of low voltage and the T waves were flattened. In patients with myxoedema who have coronary artery disease, signs of myocardial ischaemia may also be demonstrable. In the past, angina was sometimes treated by creation of a hypothyroid state in order to reduce cardiac metabolic demand. Nowadays, such patients are treated by full thyroid replacement (which lowers raised cholesterol) and management of the coronary disease, either medically alone or with surgery as the disease demands.

190 Both acute myeloid and acute lymphoblastic leukaemia are treated with regimes involving doxorubicin, which is cardiotoxic. Toxicity is dose-related, but is rare if the cumulative dose is less than 500 mg/m^2, although children can develop cardiac toxicity at lower doses. Myocardial damage is largely irreversible and presents as biventricular dilatation and reduced systolic function. Conventional treatment for heart failure is not very effective and the prognosis is poor – death usually occurs within 3 months of presentation. Withdrawal of doxorubicin does not seem to halt progression of the cardiomyopathy. Patients who receive doxorubicin require regular echocardiography or radionuclide ventriculography. Doxoribicin is stopped if there is any hint of ventricular dysfunction. The diagnosis of myocardial toxicity secondary to doxorubicin therapy can be confirmed with endomyocardial biopsy, but this is rarely necessary. Early myocardial failure soon after starting doxorubicin may resolve, but later dose-related failure does not improve. Survivors may develop a non-lethal late restrictive cardiomyopathy.

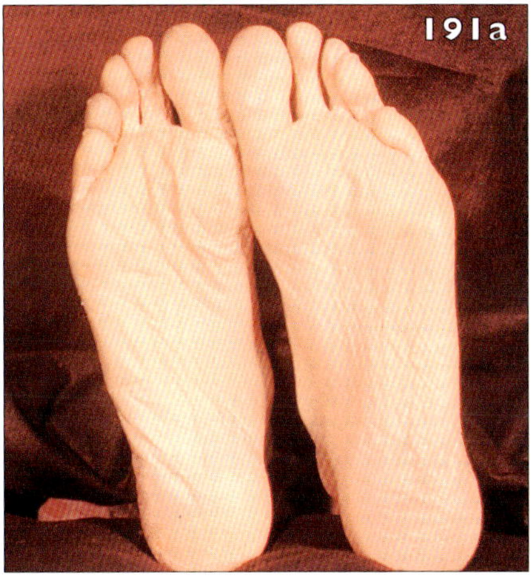

191a

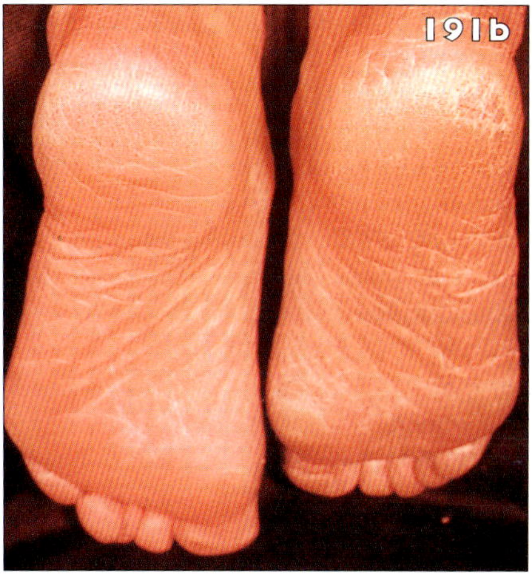

191b

191 **191a** shows the feet of a 56-year-old diabetic man after they had been elevated. **191b** shows the effect of leaving them dependent. What can you conclude?

192 This patient complained of breathlessness. Describe three classic cardiovascular physical signs which would be characteristic of this condition and explain them.

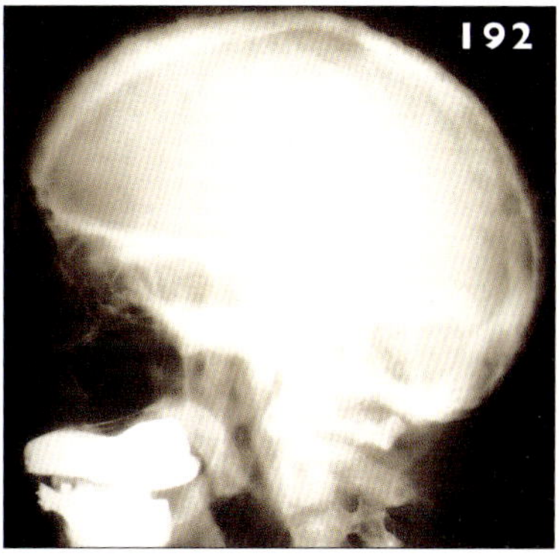

192

193 A retired woman who had undergone coronary artery bypass grafting for angina collapsed and died a week after her operation. Before her death, the ECG shown was obtained.

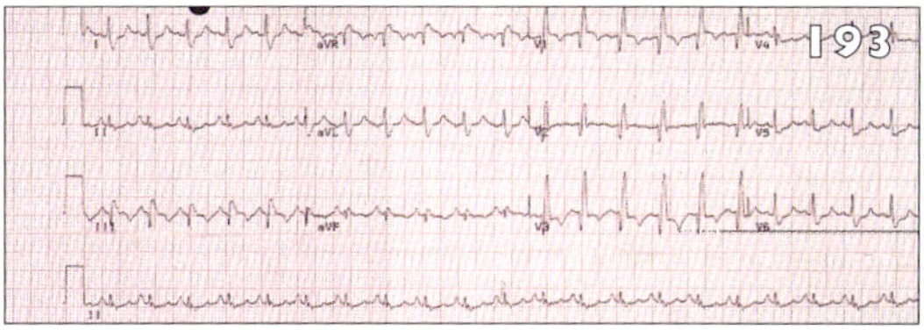

193

i. What is the likely cause of death?
ii. What measures can reduce the likelihood of this complication?

191 The marked colour change on moving the legs to a dependent position (reactionary rubor) suggests underlying peripheral vascular disease (the incidence of which is significantly greater in diabetics). This is Buerger's test. When the legs are elevated, arterial stenosis prevents adequate blood flow reaching the extremities so the leg blanches. However, when the legs are dependent, blood reaches the extremities. Initially, because of maximal small vessel dilatation due to the previous build-up of metabolic products, the legs become warm and red. However, with time, the slow rate of flow and the relative hypoxia of the tissues encourages maximal oxygen extraction to leave a higher level of deoxyhaemoglobin in the blood, which results in localised peripheral cyanosis.

192 A skull radiograph is shown. The skull vault is irregularly thickened and a number of lytic lesions can be seen, especially in the occipital region and at the vertex. The diagnosis is Paget's disease of bone. In this disorder, there is an increase in turnover of bone, primarily due to an abnormality of osteoclast activity, perhaps due to persistent infection of these cells by a paramyxovirus. If the patient is symptomatic, the usual complaint is of localised bone pain. However, arteriovenous shunting also occurs in the regions of bone dysplasia. In very severe disease this can lead to high output cardiac failure. The physical signs of the latter include a mildly raised jugular venous pressure (due to increased cardiac output), an increased pulse pressure, audible third and fourth heart sounds with or without the murmur of tricuspid regurgitation, and crepitations on auscultation of the lungs.

193 i. The clinical scenario – the fact that coronary artery bypass grafting had been performed for angina – might indicate a coronary cause for the collapse. However, examination of the ECG shows right bundle branch block, a deep S wave in standard lead I and a Q wave and inversion of the T wave in standard lead III. This 'SI,QIII,TIII' combination is a classic finding in acute pulmonary embolism.

ii. Any form of surgery is associated with a risk of deep vein thrombosis; the risk rises sharply with prolonged operations in older patients, up to 60% prevalence in the absence of any prophylaxis (however, while under cardiopulmonary bypass, patients will be heparinised due to the blood passing through the oxygenator). Pulmonary embolism is the most serious sequela of deep vein thrombosis and probably has an incidence of about 8% in cases of deep vein thrombosis. Early mobilisation post-operatively and the avoidance of prolonged bed rest (e.g. after myocardial infarction) has greatly reduced the prevalence of thrombosis. Full length anti-embolism stockings approximately halve the rate of deep vein thrombosis. Prophylactic low-dose subcutaneous heparin (5000 IU b.d. or t.i.d.) reduces the natural rate of deep vein thrombosis by about two-thirds; the effects are additive to those of anti-embolism stockings. Recently available low molecular weight fractions of heparin may have advantages with respect to the risks of excessive bleeding. Aspirin has not been shown to be beneficial.

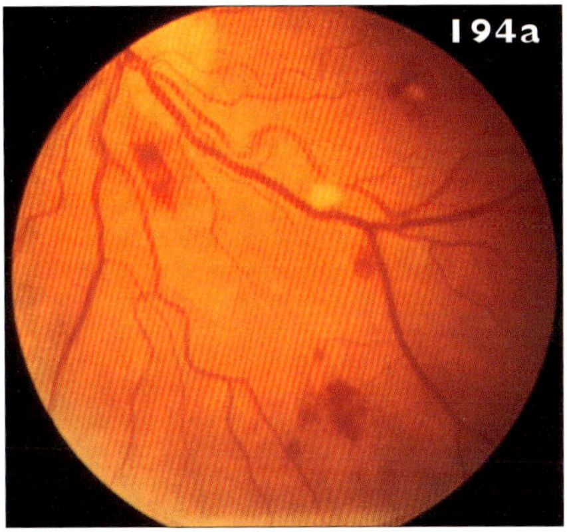

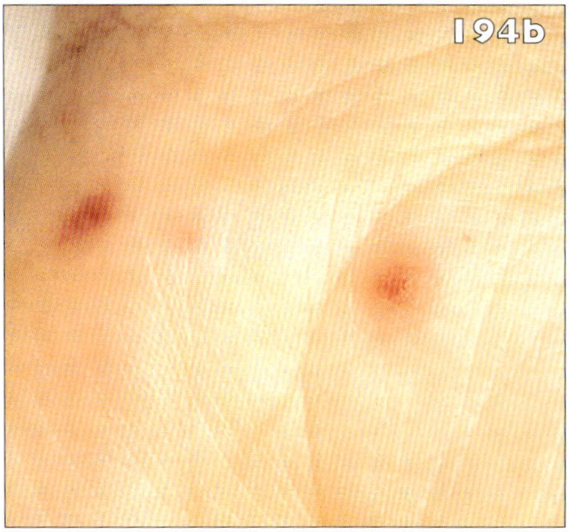

194 A man who had been feverish for the previous 3 weeks insisted on keeping a routine appointment with his optician before going to his doctor's surgery. What did the optician and the doctor see and what is the matter with this man?

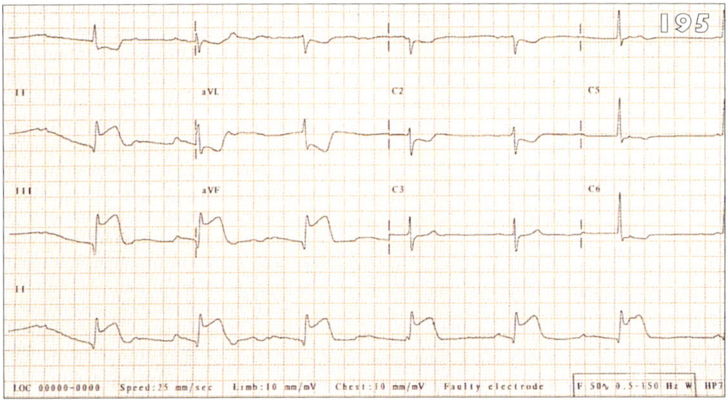

195 A 63-year-old man came to the coronary care unit with chest pain.

i. List three abnormalities on the ECG.

ii. What is the diagnosis?

iii. List four immediate steps in the management of this patient.

194 The fundus (**194a**) shows a petechial lesion with a small white central area surrounded by a red halo – a Roth spot. It is found in infective endocarditis (and in some patients with systemic lupus erythematosus). There are two equivalent lesions visible in the skin on the palmar aspect of the patient's right hand (**194b**); these are Janeway lesions. Both these lesions are probably caused by immune complex deposition. In infective endocarditis, the valvar vegetation is effectively an immunologically privileged site for the initial causative organisms, since they are protected from a granulomatous or suppurative reaction by layers of platelets and fibrin. However, the body does produce large amounts of antibody in response; it is complexes of these immunoglobin molecules which cause the lesions shown.

195 i. Three abnormalities are third-degree atrioventricular (AV) block, with a ventricular rate of 40 b.p.m., ST segment elevation in leads II, III, and aVf, and ST segment depression and T wave inversion in leads I and aVL.
ii. Acute inferior myocardial infarction complicated by third-degree AV block.
iii. Immediate management steps are: the patient should receive intravenous diamorphine to relieve pain; 40% oxygen should be instituted if there is no history of severe chronic obstructive airways disease, otherwise 24% oxygen is given; 150–300 mg of aspirin is given immediately (this is thought to save approximately 25 lives per 1000 patients); thrombolysis should be instituted as quickly as possible, which is also estimated to save a further 25 lives per 1000.

The patient should be temporarily paced to aid the circulation and avoid the risk of asystole. Second or third degree AV block can occur following a relatively small inferior myocardial infarction because the right coronary artery supplies the AV node. This is usually transient, resolving within a few days, but it may remain for 2–3 weeks. There should be bed rest for 48 hours and echocardiography to assess left ventricular function. Angiotensin-converting enzyme (ACE) inhibitors are indicated if left ventricular function is reduced, even in asymptomatic patients. Both the Survival and Ventricular Enlargement (SAVE) and the Studies of Left Ventricular Dysfunction (SOLVD) studies have demonstrated a significant reduction in morbidity and mortality when ACE inhibitors are prescribed for patients in this group. Treatment needs to be maintained for at least a year to achieve the maximum benefit. Exercise stress testing is performed to assess the risk of further cardiac events. Patients with positive exercise stress tests should be offered coronary angiography with a view to proceeding to percutaneous transluminal angioplasty or coronary artery bypass grafting, depending on the severity of the coronary artery disease. All patients below the age of 60 years should have coronary angiography for prognostic purposes. Risk factors for further ischaemic events should be addressed; these include weight reduction in overweight patients, advice regarding smoking and a low lipid diet, control of co-existing diabetes and hypertension, and the management of hyperlipidaemia.

196 The ECG shown was obtained during an episode of chest pain in a 46-year-old man who had frequent and severe anginal attacks, which were not very responsive to treatment with either long-acting nitrates or beta-blockers. His coronary angiogram showed moderate two-vessel coronary disease – a 70% proximal left circumflex and a 60% mid-right coronary arterial stenosis.

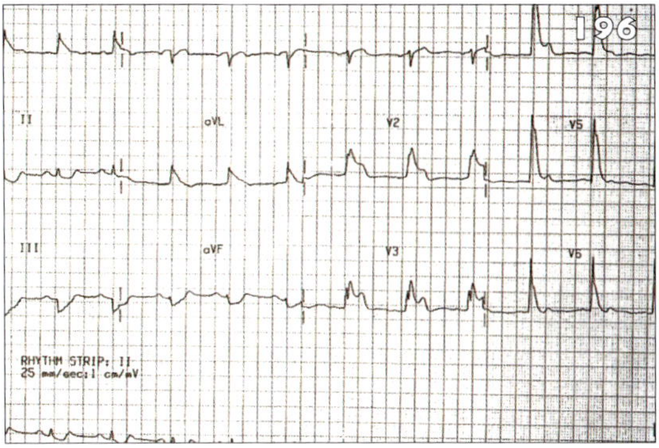

i. What does the ECG show?
ii. What is the underlying problem?
iii. How would you treat it?

197 A 30-year-old man underwent a routine medical to obtain a licence to drive heavy vehicles.

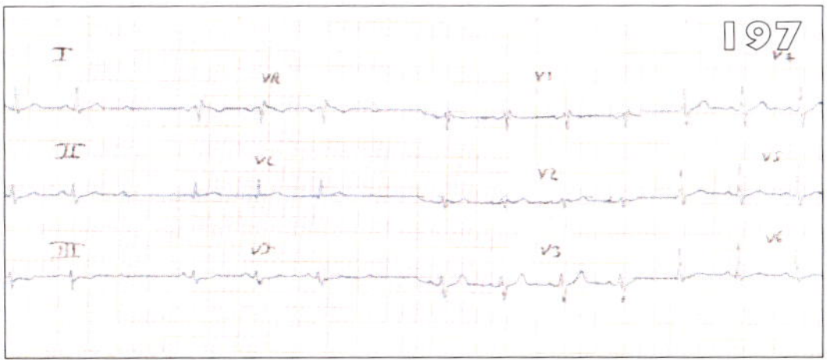

i. What is the ECG diagnosis?
ii. What is the prognosis?
iii. Should the man be denied a licence on medical grounds?

198 This 55-year-old man was being monitored for 24 hours after admission with unstable angina. What does the ECG show?

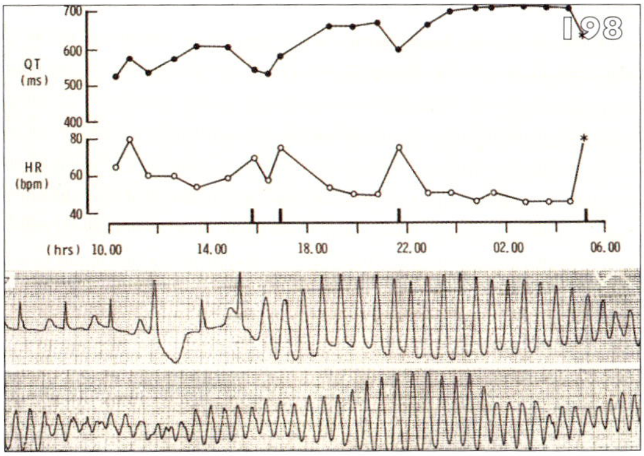

196 i. The ECG shows convex ST segment elevation in the anterior chest leads.
ii. This is a case of variant (Prinzmetal's) angina.
iii. Variant angina is characterised by frequent and severe episodes of angina that usually occur at rest; the accompanying ECG changes are typically those of convex-upward ST segment elevation. Angiography shows either normal or only moderately diseased coronary arteries, with usually no flow-limiting epicardial arterial stenoses. Provocation tests to demonstrate coronary spasm, e.g. by forced hyperventilation or by intravenous (or rarely intracoronary) ergonovine, may be of diagnostic value. In the case in question, calcium antagonist drugs have not been used and would be the medical treatment of first choice. The underlying cause of the arterial predisposition towards constriction is probably abnormal endothelial function, with a failure of NO production. This is consistent with coronary spasm being more frequent at sites of pre-existing atheroma or arterial injury.

197 i. The ECG shows an rSR´ complex in leads V1 and V2, i.e. the leads most oriented towards the right ventricle. However, the overall QRS complex duration is not prolonged beyond 100 ms. The diagnosis is therefore partial right bundle branch block (RBBB). The reason for this M-shaped complex is that only after depolarisation of the septum (from left to right, producing the initial r wave in V1) and depolarisation of the left ventricular free wall (from right to left, producing the S wave in V1) does right ventricular depolarisation occur. When it does, it is due to the anomalous spread of depolarisation through the right ventricular free wall. This delayed left-to-right depolarisation produces the R´ wave.
ii. The outlook for partial RBBB (in the absence of structural heart defects such as atrial septal defect) is entirely normal.
iii. There is no reason for this man to be denied a licence.

198 The trace shows an 'R on T' ectopic beat followed by ventricular tachycardia. What is actually happening here is that a ventricular extrasystole is occurring with a very short coupling interval from the preceding T wave. It occurs during the vulnerable phase of repolarisation of the ventricular myocardium, when degeneration into ventricular fibrillation is a significant risk. The very fact that a ventricular extrasystole can occur with so short a coupling interval indicates that the responsible myocardium is abnormal (in this case due to myocardial ischaemia). The refractory period of this myocardium is abnormally short; this is the substrate for the development of and propagation of ventricular tachycardia and fibrillation.

199 A 60-year-old miner, who had retired early for medical reasons, died. The specimen shown was obtained at autopsy.
i. What do you see?
ii. Suggest a diagnosis.

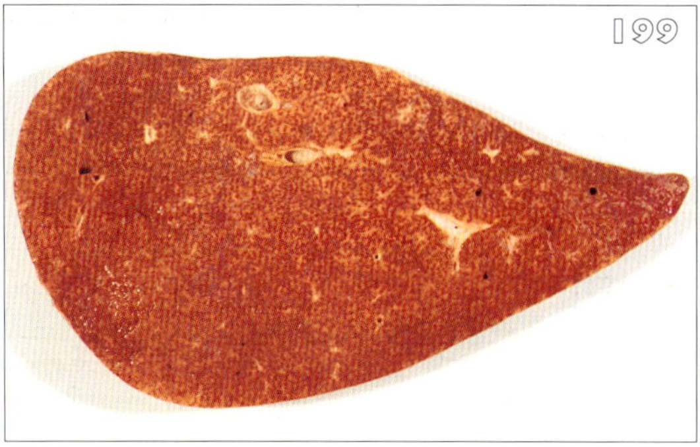

200 Cardiac catheterisation was performed on a 58-year-old woman, because of a 6-month history of worsening fatigue and shortness of breath. The pressures measured are shown (right). What is the diagnosis?

Chamber	*Pressure (mmHg)*
Pulmonary capillary wedge (mean)	32
Pulmonary artery	45/25
Right ventricle	45/13
Right atrium	a, 10; v, 8
Left ventricle	150/20
Aorta	150/40

201 A 50-year-old man developed acute chest pain, severe nausea, and sweating. He died before admission to hospital.
i. What is this investigation?
ii. What does it reveal?

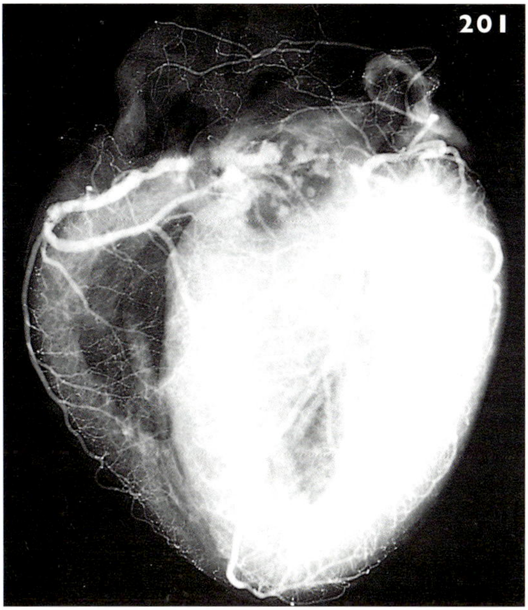

199 i. and **ii.** This 60-year-old miner had, in the course of his work and in conjunction with his cigarette smoking, developed coal worker's pneumoconiosis. In this disorder, small dust particles (2–5 µm diameter) are retained in the small airways and provoke fibrosis. Due both to the dust-induced fibrosis and the loss of lung tissue and pulmonary vasoconstriction, all features of chronic obstructive airways disease, there is a gradual increase in right ventricular afterload. Pulmonary hypertension leads to right ventricular hypertrophy, the degree of which is positively correlated with the extent of pulmonary arterial medial hypertrophy. The pulmonary hypertension is usually only moderate and right ventricular failure – cor pulmonale – only occurs when there is also alveolar hypoventilation with carbon dioxide retention, respiratory acidosis, metabolic alkalosis, and fluid retention. In other words, it is 'blue bloaters' and not 'pink puffers' who tend to develop right ventricular failure. The chronic rise in venous pressure leads to congestion of hepatic venules with centrilobular necrosis. This causes the alternating dark and light banding which can be seen on this macroscopic section from the liver – the so-called 'nutmeg' liver.

200 The pulmonary capillary wedge pressure (and by inference left atrial pressure) is raised at 32 mmHg, pulmonary artery pressure is also raised at 45/25 mmHg, as is the right ventricular pressure (45/13 mmHg); there is no gradient across the pulmonary valve. The left ventricular systolic pressure is normal, but the end-diastolic pressure is elevated at 20 mmHg. The left ventricular end-diastolic pressure and the pulmonary artery wedge pressure do not equalise, but there is a gradient of 12 mmHg across the mitral valve, i.e. the patient has mitral stenosis. The right atrial pressures are slightly elevated and a degree of tricuspid regurgitation is present (see *Appendix* for normal values). Although there is no significant gradient across the aortic valve, the systemic pulse pressure is abnormally wide. The diagnoses are therefore aortic regurgitation and mitral stenosis, with a minor degree of tricuspid regurgitation.

201 i. A post-mortem coronary angiogram is shown.
ii. The heart is hypertrophied. The injection of the coronary arteries shows an occlusion of the proximal right coronary artery. The clinical history of acute chest pain and 'vagal' symptoms of severe nausea and sweating point to a diagnosis of a (fatal) inferior myocardial infarction. This is consistent with the pathological anatomic findings in the right coronary artery. The reason for the association of 'vagal' symptoms with inferior infarction relates to the selectively more extensive vagal innervation of the posteroinferior aspect of the heart as compared to the anterior wall. Reflex activation of vagal efferents occurs in response to increased vagal afferent activity from the territory of the infarct. As far as can be discerned, the left anterior descending and left circumflex coronary arteries are free from significant disease. The myocardial hypertrophy may be an indicator of previous hypertensive heart disease, which would also be a risk factor for coronary artery disease.

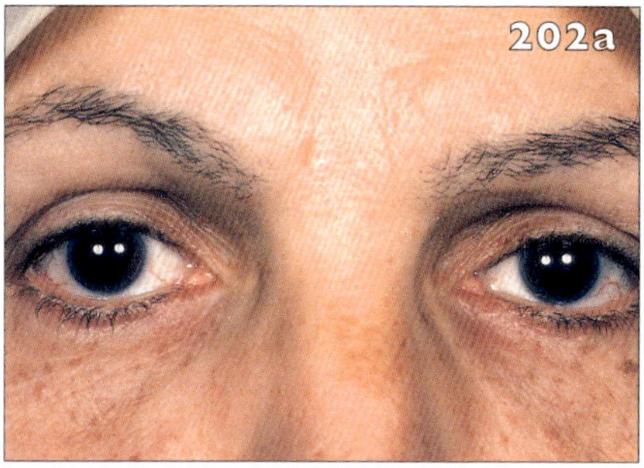
202a

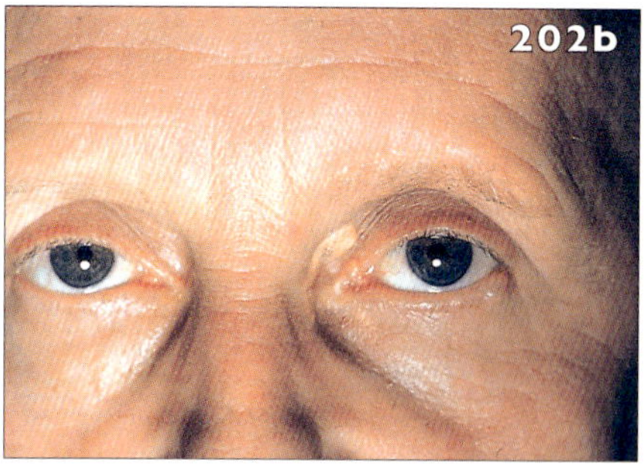
202b

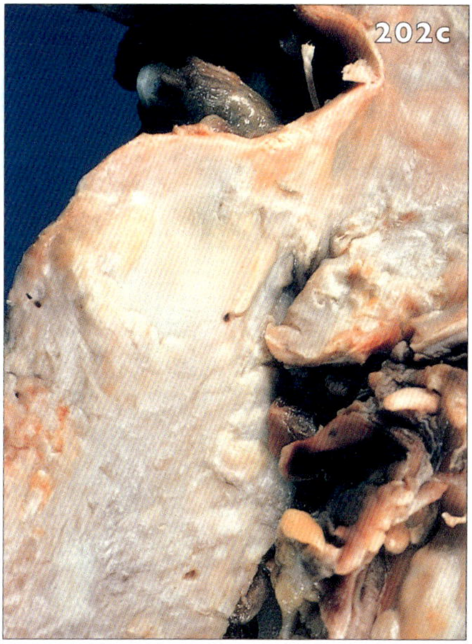
202c

202 **i.** What physical signs can you see?
ii. What post-mortem findings can you see in **202c** from a relative of the people shown in **202a** and **202b**?
iii. Suggest an underlying diagnosis.
iv. What management advice would you give these (asymptomatic) patients?

203 A 24-year-old woman, previously noted to have 'a murmur', was sent for further investigations.
i. What is this investigation?
ii. What does it show?
iii. What other key physical sign would you expect to find?

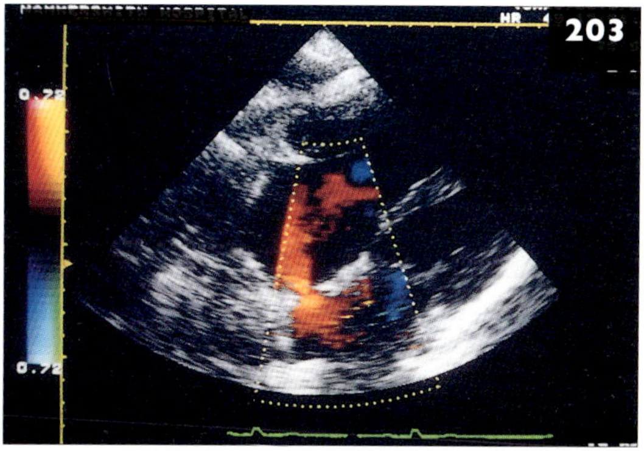
203

202 i. 202a and **202b** show, respectively, arcus senilis and xanthelasmata.
ii. 202c shows extensive atheroma, including ulcerated plaques in the aorta and coronary arteries.
iii. This severity of atheroma points to an underlying dyslipidaemia and the diagnosis is familial hypercholesterolaemia. The risk of coronary events is substantially increased if total cholesterol >5.2 mmol/l, triglycerides >3.0 mmol/l, or LDL/HDL ratio >3.5.
iv. The woman should undergo a cardiovascular work-up, including a 12-lead ECG, exercise treadmill test and, depending upon the findings, diagnostic coronary angiography, as well as a detailed lipid profile. In terms of management, the first stage is dietary manipulation in the form of a diet low in animal fat. Subsequently, drugs of value include resins (e.g. cholestyramine, although it may be hard for adequate doses to be tolerable), nicotinic acid (which probably acts via a reduction in mobilisation of free fatty acids from adipose tissue), fibrates (e.g. gemfibrizol and bezafibrate, both of which raise HDL and lower LDL, total cholesterol, and triglycerides), and the statins (drugs which inhibit HMGCoA reductase and raise the number of LDL receptors). The statins are the drugs of choice in pure hypercholesterolaemia.

203 i. The investigation is a colour flow Doppler study. This is a subcostal four chamber view.
ii. It shows flow across the atrial septum, from the left atrium to the right, suggestive of an atrial septal defect (ASD). Two-dimensional echocardiography not only enables the demonstration of ASD, but also allows differentiation of the anatomical type of septal defect. In the case of an ostium primum defect (partial atrioventricular canal), no atrial septal material is attached to the ventricular septum and the insertions of the mitral and tricuspid valves are level. Full details of the different types of complete atrioventricular canal defects are visualised in this view. In contrast, in the secundum type defect shown here, the defect is more posterior and higher, so the normal Z insertion of the atrioventricular valves is preserved. Colour flow Doppler can increase the value of the investigation by demonstrating the direction of flow across the septal defect and thus document the direction of shunting. Continuous-wave Doppler echocardiography can then be employed to quantify the velocity of the jets. The pulmonary and systemic flow rates can also be derived.
iii. The classic physical sign in this condition is fixed splitting of the second heart sound. (The left-to-right intracardiac shunt decreases on inspiration. There is a lack of the normal prolongation of right ventricular systole and reduction of left ventricular systole on inspiration, so that the normal respiratory variation of the second heart sound does not occur.)

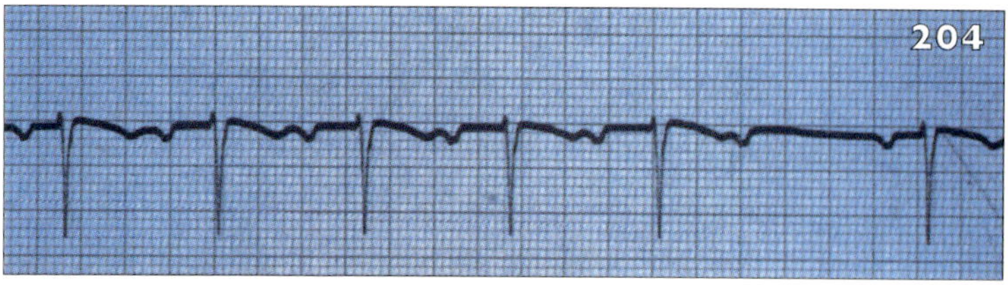

204 What is the ECG diagnosis?

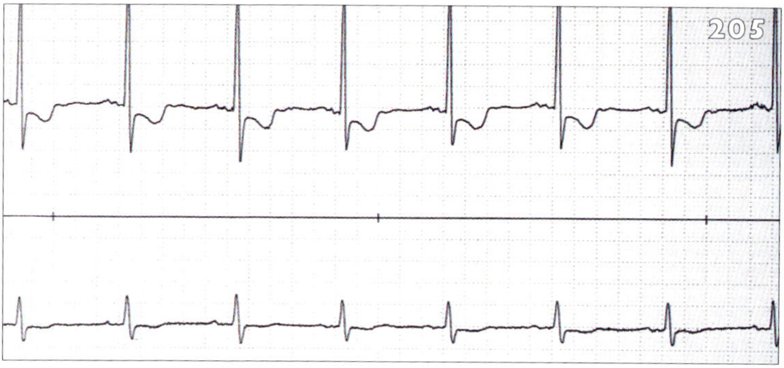

205 A 56-year-old man with a previous myocardial infarction complains of infrequent (< twice a week) episodes of angina. He underwent a period of ambulatory ECG monitoring in the course of which he experienced no chest pain.

i. What abnormality does the ECG strip show?

ii. What is the significance of this finding?

206 This is a chest radiograph of a 77-year-old patient who presented with breathlessness, weight gain, constipation and increasing memory loss. What is the probable cause of the abnormality on the chest radiograph?

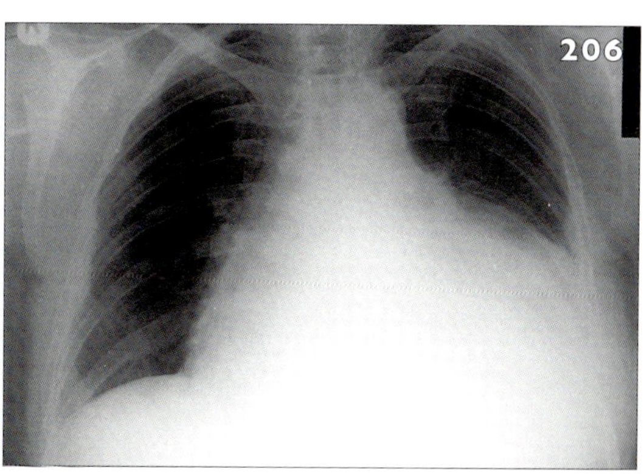

204 The diagnosis is Mobitz Type 1 atrioventricular (AV) block or Wenkebach AV block. This is a form of second-degree block in which delay in AV conduction increases with each atrial impulse until an atrial impulse fails to be conducted to the ventricles. This is seen as a progressive increase in the PR interval until a P wave fails to conduct and is therefore not followed by a QRS complex. After this has occurred AV conduction is restored and the whole process begins again. Mobitz Type I AV block can be benign and in young people is attributed to a high vagal tone. It can also be secondary to ischaemic heart disease, particularly following inferior myocardial infarction when it may be a transient phenomenon, or to cardiac conduction tissue disease. In these situations the prognosis is not as good as was once believed, so if patients are symptomatic they should have a permanent pacemaker implanted, which not only ameliorates the symptoms but also returns life expectancy to normal.

205 **i.** The ECG strips shows several episodes of ST segment depression, indicating myocardial ischaemia even though no chest pain was reported (i.e. the ischaemia was silent).
ii. Ambulatory electrocardiographic monitoring has been of great importance in the identification and research of reversible silent myocardial ischaemia. Clinically, silent myocardial ischaemia is associated with a poor prognosis, e.g. after unstable angina or myocardial infarction. It has been presumed in patients in whom sudden cardiac death is the first presentation of coronary artery disease, since silent ischaemia has been found during exercise in cardiac arrest survivors and in patients with life-threatening arrhythmias. The pathophysiological basis of silent ischaemia has not been established, but it might be milder than painful ischaemia in patients experiencing both. The higher incidence in diabetics has implicated autonomic neuropathy in the silence of the ischaemia. Finally, altered central nervous handling of messages from the heart, possibly mediated through the brain's opiate systems, might explain the phenomenon.

206 There is gross cardiomegaly, which may be secondary to a pericardial effusion or a dilated cardiomyopathy. The history of breathlessness, weight gain, constipation and increasing memory loss taken in an elderly patient with this chest radiograph should raise the suspicion of hypothyroidism, although, in the elderly, such symptoms are common, even in the absence of an underlying illness. Thyroxine (T4) and thyroid-stimulating hormone (TSH) levels must be checked in all elderly patients with these symptoms. T4 is usually low and TSH is always elevated in hypothyroidism. Cardiac manifestations of hypothyroidism are secondary to a low metabolic rate and a low cardiac output. Sinus bradycardia, low pulse pressure, congestive cardiac failure, pericardial effusions and coronary artery disease all occur. The ECG demonstrates bradycardia, low voltage complexes and, occasionally, conduction defects. Management requires replacement with thyroxine, starting at the lowest dose of 25 μg daily and increasing the dose every 4 to 6 weeks. Over-rapid replacement can lead to angina, atrial fibrillation and worsening of cardiac failure (see **189**).

207 The traces in **207b** were obtained from a 67-year-old man who had an acute anterior myocardial infarction 36 hours previously (**207a** was obtained from a normal control). (ADC, apexcardiogram; PA, pulmonary area; MA, mitral area; MF, medium frequency filter; LF, low frequency filter.) Explain the differences between the traces and suggest some abnormal physical signs that you might be able to elicit.

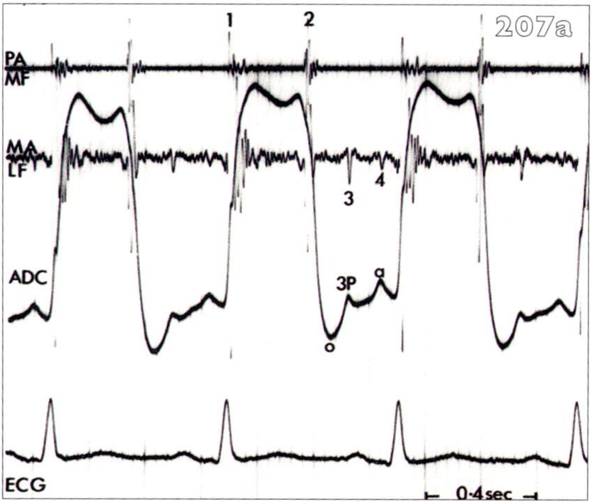

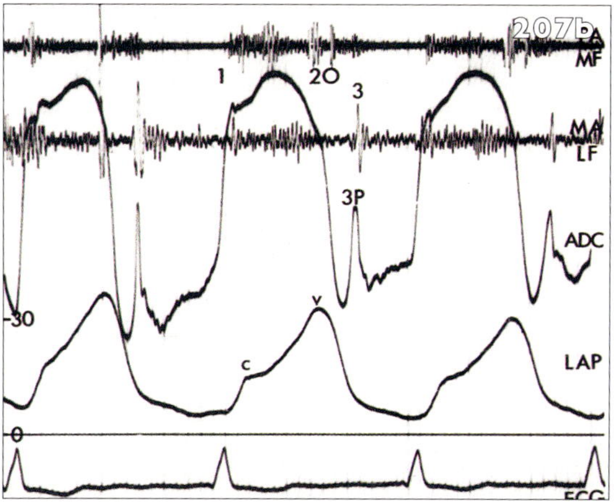

208 **i.** What is the ECG diagnosis?
ii. What are the possible causes of this type of arrhythmia?
iii. What are the possible management strategies?
iv. How could further episodes of the arrhythmia be prevented?

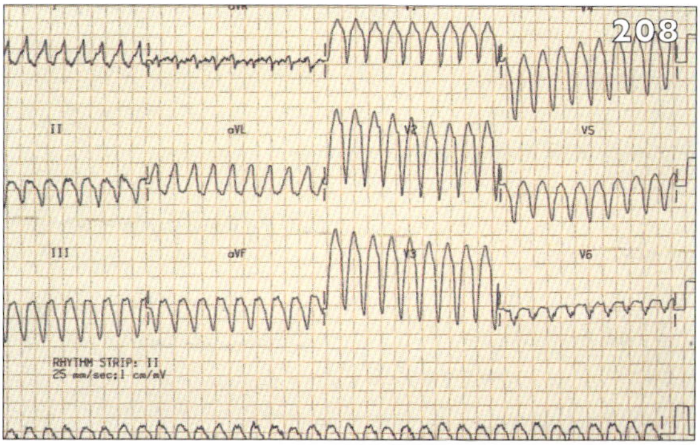

207 The traces show an apexcardiogram, i.e. traces which, via a pressure transducer applied to the palpable apical impulse, describe the motion of the cardiac apex through the cardiac cycle. The normal trace (**207a**) can be divided into the following phases: A, a small outward deflection due to atrial contraction; a sharp upstroke with the onset of ventricular systole; the upstroke ends at point E, the onset of left ventricular ejection. As the ventricular volume falls, the apical movement is inward; more rapid inward movement occurs around S2 as the nadir or O point is reached (this also corresponds to the lowest left ventricular pressure). Outward movement recommences after the O point and ceases with the end of the rapid filling wave (point F); this point is coincident with the normal third heart sound. The cycle is completed by the slow filling phase which precedes atrial contraction.

After myocardial infarction, the left ventricle is generally stiffer than in health and a more forceful atrial contraction is required (an enhanced A on the apexcardiogram), resulting in a clinically audible and palpable fourth heart sound. Left ventricular damage causes the initial outward movement during systole to be slower and less forceful, causing a reduction in the E wave.

208 **i.** The ECG shows ventricular tachycardia – a broad complex tachycardia with QRS complexes exceeding 120 ms. There is extreme axis shift and concordance in all the chest leads. It is difficult to see dissociated P waves.
ii. The most common cause of ventricular tachycardia is myocardial ischaemia, but acute myocardial infarction can also cause it. Ventricular tachycardia is a recognised complication of scar-tissue formation following myocardial infarction, in which case it occurs several weeks after the infarction. Cardiomyopathies are the second most common cause of ventricular tachycardia. Other causes include myocarditis, drug abuse with tricyclic antidepressants, mitral valve prolapse, valvar heart disease, as a complication of late repair of Fallot's tetralogy, and in right ventricular dysplasia.
iii. If the arrhythmia is sustained and causes cardiac arrest or profound hypotension, immediate cardioversion is necessary. If the arrhythmia is well-tolerated, then lignocaine is the first-line drug given. Amiodarone is a useful second-line drug with no negative inotropic effect; however, its onset of action can take hours rather than minutes. Pacing is occasionally used, particularly when drugs are ineffective and repeated cardioversion is not practical due to recurrent episodes of ventricular tachycardia.
iv. Further episodes could be prevented by: drugs (flecainide, sotalol, disopyramide, and amiodarone – anti-tachycardia pacing devices; surgery – the arrhythmogenic focus can be isolated by ventricular mapping and surgically excised (a high-risk procedure) and catheter ablation, which is being carried out with increasing frequency. Prior to catheter ablation, an electrophysiology study is performed. In this, the arrhythmia is provoked by ventricular stimulation using catheters introduced into the heart via the femoral arterial and venous route. The culprit area is then ablated by delivering a high-current shock via an electrode catheter.

209 A 78-year-old woman, who had complained of feeling unwell for 6 months, was found dead by a neighbour. A post-mortem was performed and the disease found (**209a** shows the gross appearance and **209b** the microscopic) was considered responsible for death.

i. What was the disease?

ii. Give three extra-cardiac presentations.

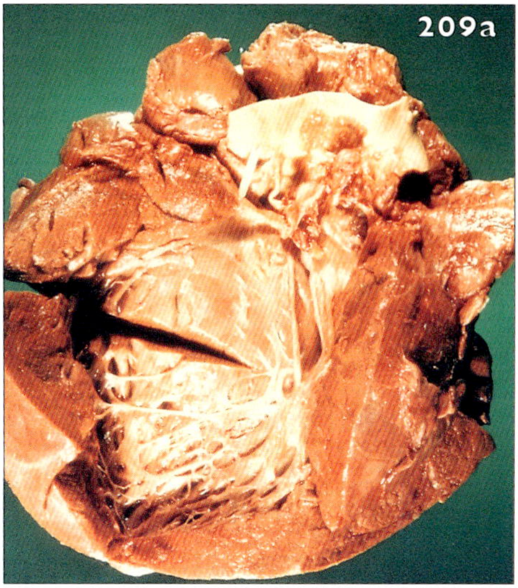

209a

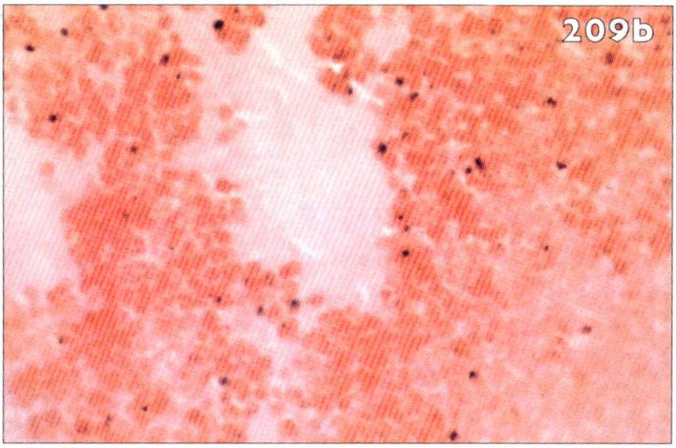

209b

210 A 60-year-old man presented with acute, severe chest pain and the investigation shown was performed as a matter of urgency.

i. What is the investigation?

ii. What does it show?

iii. Is this the most appropriate way to investigate this problem?

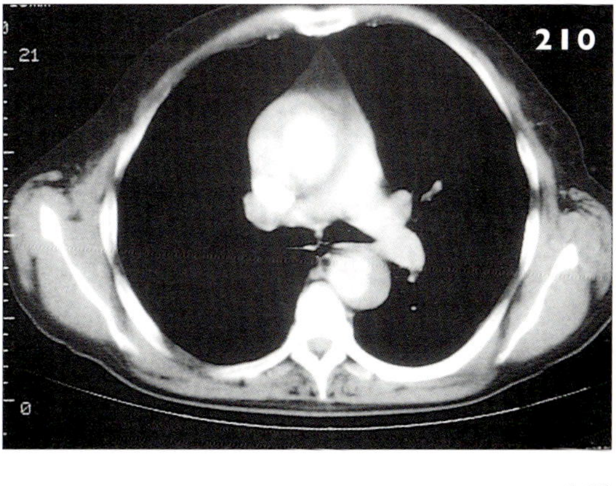

210

209 i. 209a shows the gross pathology and **209b** the microscopy of vegetations from this woman who had infective endocarditis. Various aspects of the question are instructive with respect to the presentation and clinical features of this disease today. In contrast to a century ago, when sepsis was the leading cause of endocarditis, most cases of native valve endocarditis now occur in older patients with degenerating valves. The annual incidence is probably about 2/100,000 of the UK population, with a male preponderance due to the higher incidence of aortic valve disease in men and decreasing incidence of rheumatic heart disease, which was more common in women. The presentation can be rather non-specific (e.g. malaise, fatigue, anorexia and weight loss) and the diagnosis is often not considered. Fever is almost invariable, but apart from infection with virulent organisms (usually staphylococci), severe pyrexia and rigors are unusual.

ii. Besides the detection of new murmurs and signs of heart failure, extra-cardiac presentations of the disease are important clues to the underlying disease. These include fever, anaemia, arthralgia, splenomegaly, emboli to the retina, brain, kidney, spleen and gut, generalised vasculitis, toxic encephalopathy, retinal haemorrhages (e.g. Roth spots), Osler's nodes and Janeway lesions. Metastatic abscesses can present via continuing fever. In the case of cardiac abscesses, there may be new conduction defects on the ECG. Pericarditis is also a recognised complication.

210 i. The investigation shown is a transverse CT scan of the thorax.

ii. It shows a dissecting aneurysm of the aorta involving the ascending and descending aorta, the classification is therefore Type A (or, according to the DeBakey classification, Type I).

iii. This question complements **42**. As indicated there, in the immediate investigation of a suspected dissection of the aorta, both echocardiography and CT scanning of the thorax can be readily available and have the advantage of being non-invasive. The extent of dissection visible on trans-thoracic echo (TTE) may be limited, but much more information is quickly obtained by transoesophageal echo (TOE). CT images, which can be enhanced by the use of intravenous contrast, can define the origin of the dissection and its extent. Aortography is used decreasingly and may not show the lesion at all.

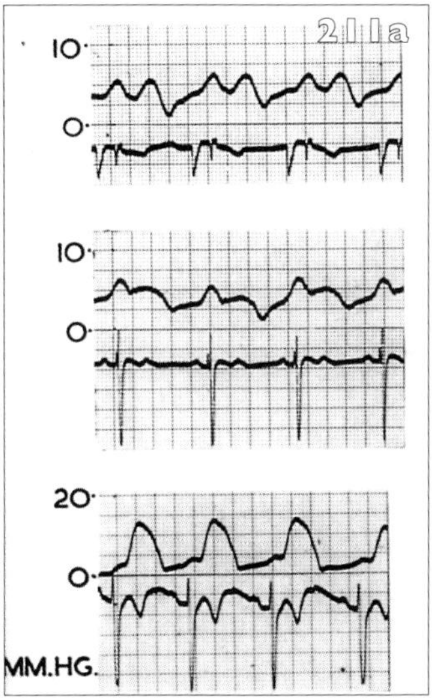

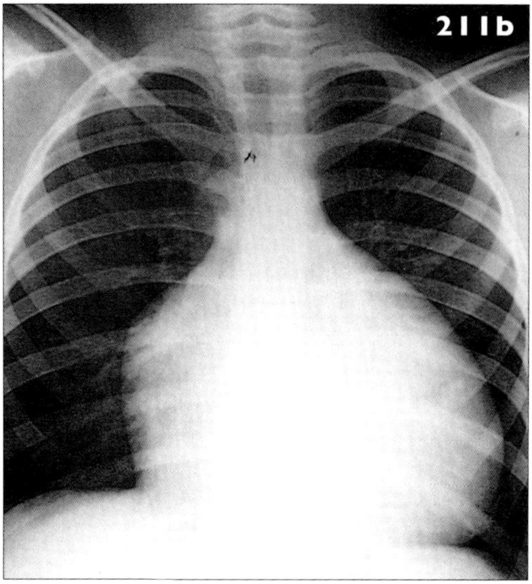

211 An electrophysiological study of a 20-year-old male patient who presented with palpitations and breathlessness produced the wave morphologies shown in **211a** (top, high right atrium; middle, low right atrium; bottom, right ventricle). A chest radiograph of the same condition is shown in **211b**.
i. What is the underlying diagnosis?
ii. Name a commonly associated arrhythmia.
iii. What is it due to?

212 An asymptomatic 28-year-old man, whose brother had died suddenly at the age of 18, had been referred for investigation after a new family doctor had examined him for an incidental mild complaint and had found a cardiac murmur. The young doctor who had seen the patient ordered an exercise treadmill test during which the tracing shown was produced.

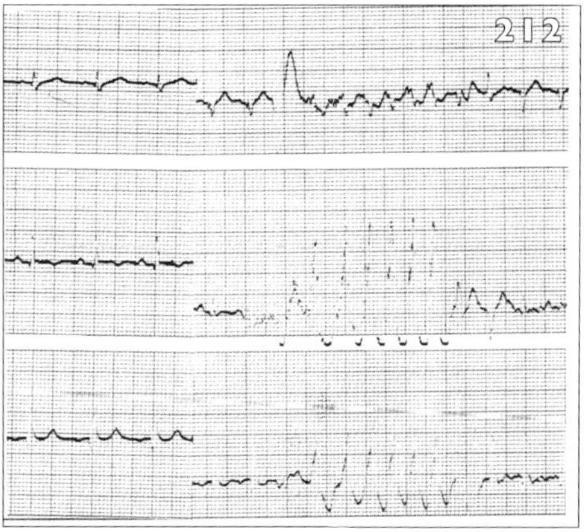

i. What does the ECG show?
ii. Give the most likely underlying diagnosis?
iii. Was it a good idea to have ordered the exercise test?

211 i. The wave morphologies shown in the middle trace of **211a** show a right atrial pressure wave accompanied by a right ventricular electrocardiographic pattern. The underlying diagnosis is Ebstein's anomaly. The underlying lesion is a downwards displacement of the proximal attachments of one or more tricuspid valve leaflets into the right ventricular cavity. The valve leaflets may be absent, fused, or perforated with abnormal chordae; it is usually the posterior and septal leaflets which are displaced down into the ventricular inlet. The anterior leaflet is normally attached, but redundant and sail-like. Tricuspid regurgitation may be absent or marked. The other pathophysiological consequences of the anomaly can be seen to follow straightforwardly. There is impairment of right ventricular function, the extent of which depends upon the amount of right ventricle which has been 'atrialised'.
ii. and **iii.** Rhythm disturbances, usually atrial flutter, are a recognised feature. Atrioventricular tachycardia is frequently due to accessory pathways, often multiple, which are associated with at least 10% of cases of Ebstein's anomaly.
iii. The pre-excitation is usually mediated by a right-sided accessory pathway and is potentially dangerous because of the tendency of the dilated right atrium to develop flutter, with the risk of 1:1 atrioventricular conduction which may be followed by cardiac arrest due to ventricular fibrillation. In the management of Ebstein's anomaly, the associated Wolff–Parkinson–White syndrome is not usually amenable to radiofrequency ablation because of the multiple pathways involved.

212 i. At rest, the ECG shows T wave inversion in the middle trace and a Q wave in the lower trace. On exercise, an R on T ectopic beat occurred and was followed by ventricular tachycardia.
ii. The underlying diagnosis is hypertrophic cardiomyopathy (HCM), of which the man's brother had died suddenly in his teens. Examination of this patient revealed a late systolic murmur due to the gradient across the ventricular outflow tract.
iii. In HCM, exercise testing is prognostically of value to assess effort tolerance and blood pressure response to exercise. The former is further advanced by respiratory monitoring at the same time, particularly since maximal oxygen consumption and ventilatory capacity are often reduced, even in asymptomatic cases. The blood pressure response to exercise is abnormal in over 30% of cases, with falls in systolic pressure at peak exercise, possibly due to a disturbance of baroreflex control. The ST segment changes found during exercise testing are difficult to interpret in view of the resting ECG abnormality.

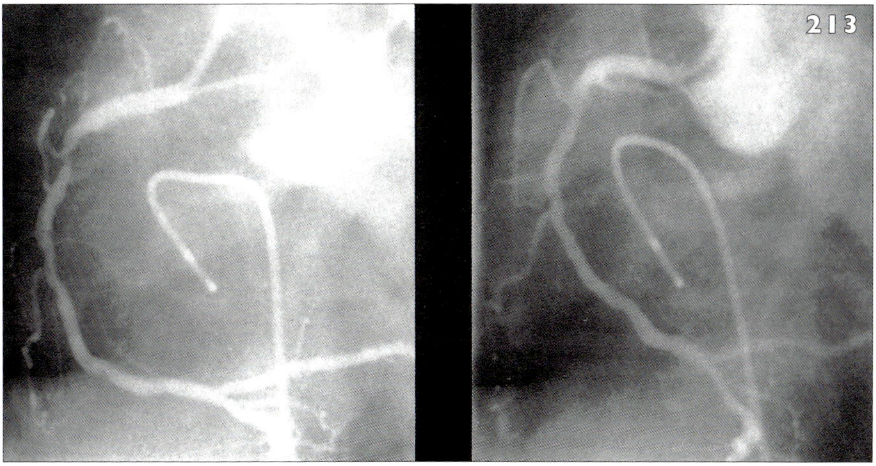

213 What do these images demonstrate?

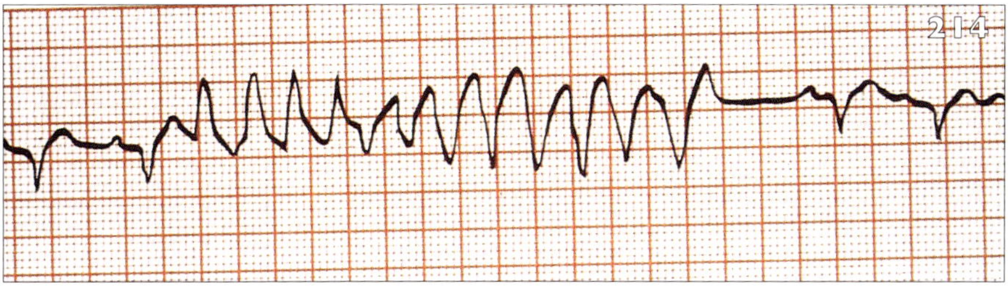

214 A 70-year-old patient collapsed in the waiting area of the heart failure clinic. He recovered after a few seconds of unconsciousness and was admitted to the cardiac care unit for monitoring. The trace shown was obtained during a subsequent dizzy spell.

i. Give the diagnosis.

ii. What is the most likely underlying cause?

iii. What is the treatment of choice?

213 The angiograms show a successful percutaneous angioplasty to the mid portion of the right coronary artery. Percutaneous coronary artery angioplasty (PTCA) is performed using local anaesthetic. The femoral approach is most commonly used, although the procedure can be carried out via the brachial route. It is an effective form of treatment in patients with ischaemic heart disease who have refractory angina despite drug therapy and in patients with significant coronary artery disease who are not considered fit for coronary artery bypass surgery. Multiple stenoses can now be negotiated during the same procedure. Discrete, short, non-calcified lesions are ideal. The mortality rate is approximately 0.5%, but slightly higher in patients with multi-vessel disease or unstable angina. Restenosis occurs in approximately 25% of cases, usually within the first 6 months. No drug therapy has so far been shown to reduce the rate of restenosis. Patients who continue to smoke and those with diabetes mellitus have a higher incidence of restenosis. The overall mortality is similar to that from coronary artery bypass grafting. PTCA has the advantage of being much less invasive and requires merely overnight hospital stay when performed electively. Patients with PTCA are more likely to develop recurrence of symptoms and require anti-anginal medication or repeat angioplasty as compared with patients who undergo coronary surgery. In general, patients with single-vessel coronary artery disease are given PTCA. Patients with two-vessel disease are also considered if the lesions are not complicated, calcified, or too proximal in the left anterior descending coronary artery. Patients with important three-vessel coronary artery disease or a left main stem stenosis are usually managed surgically.

214 **i.** The trace shows a polymorphic ventricular tachycardia with a gradual shift in axis over the course of a number of beats. It is torsades de pointes.
ii. There are congenital and acquired disorders associated with torsades de pointes. It is frequently associated with prolongation of the QT interval, which may be due to hereditary disorders, such as Jervell and Lange-Nielsen syndrome and the Romano–Ward syndrome (see **219**), or to acquired causes, such as anti-arrhythmic drugs, bradycardia (due to various causes, including head injuries and strokes, particularly in certain cerebral regions), or hypokalaemia. In the context of the question, the patient is 70 years old. This argues against a congenital long QT syndrome and, as he is attending a heart failure clinic, this makes diuretic usage with consequent hypokalaemia likely.
iii. The management of torsades de pointes can be divided into acute and preventative measures, in addition to removal of the primary causes of acquired long QT syndromes. The use of magnesium sulphate bolus and infusion is often effective, as is temporary or permanent pacing (ideally atrial) or isoprenaline infusion. Correction of electrolyte abnormalities is mandatory. Drugs which promote QT prolongation (e.g. sotalol) should be withdrawn and alternatives employed. For the primary long QT syndromes, beta-blocker prophylaxis is of value and there is an increasing role for automatic implanted cardioverter–defibrillators. Unlike in acquired long QT syndromes, isoprenaline is contraindicated in congenital forms.

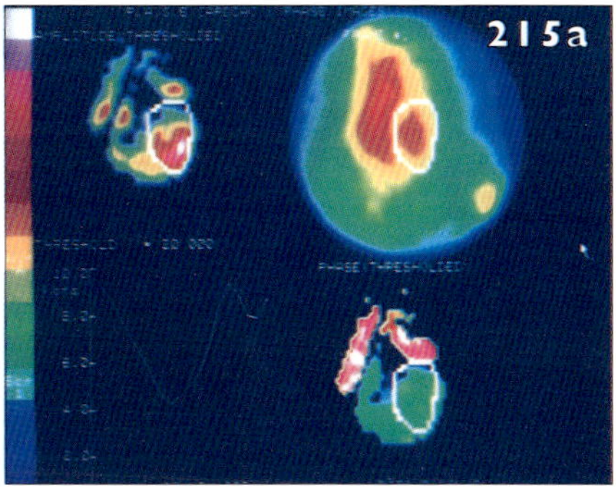

215a

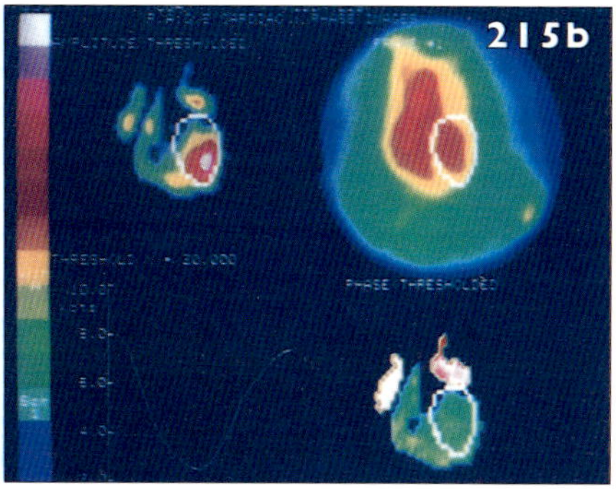

215b

215 A patient with chest pain, but in whom coronary arteriography had shown normal coronary arteries, was referred for further assessment of her ventricular function. During earlier testing, an ischaemic-looking ECG response to exercise had been obtained, but there was no evidence of left bundle branch block, either at rest or on exertion.

i. What is the investigation?

ii. What result would you anticipate under the circumstances described?

216 A 28-year-old postgraduate student from Hong Kong was admitted complaining of chest pain and vague abdominal discomfort over 3 months and weight loss over 9 months. A day later she had a stroke, which on CT scanning appeared to be due to a cerebral infarct. Two days later she died. What was the diagnosis and what happened?

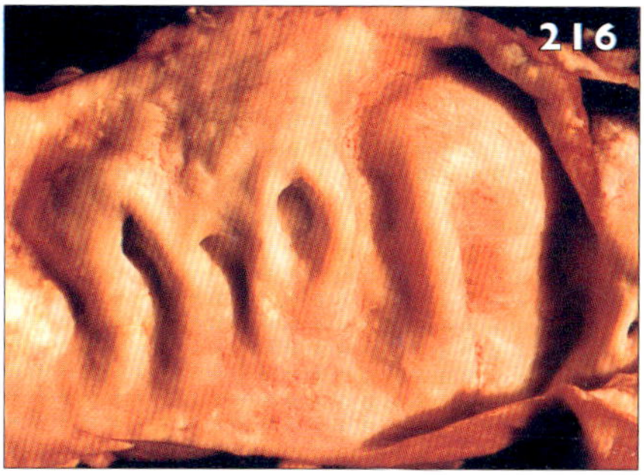

216

217 A 21-year-old woman was admitted to hospital with a 6-month history of increasing palpitations associated with dyspnoea. Since the age of 18 years she had been seeing a neurologist for difficulty with walking up stairs. Her father died suddenly when 30 years of age, but the cause of death was never ascertained. On examination she appeared well. Her heart rate was 102 b.p.m. irregularly irregular, blood pressure was 110/60 mmHg and her JVP was not elevated. On auscultation of the precordium, her heart sounds were normal and there was a pan-systolic murmur, heard loudest at the apex. Her chest was clear, but neurological examination demonstrated weakness of both lower limbs. An ECG revealed atrial fibrillation with small voltage complexes and a chest radiograph showed an enlarged cardiac shadow. Thyroid function tests were normal. What is the diagnosis?

215 **i.** This is a radionuclide multi-gated ventriculogram (MUGA), a technique in which the heart is scanned after 99m-technetium-labelled red cells (the patient's own) are injected intravenously. This method used to be the 'gold standard' for the non-invasive assessment of ventricular function and it still is for the acquisition of ejection fractions for research studies. Ejection fractions can be assessed at rest (**215a**) and after pharmacological stress, such as intravenous dipyridamole (**215b**) or adenosine, or after exercise, for evidence of ischaemia. Use of single photon emission computed tomography (SPECT) for the ventriculography, rather than planar tomography, significantly improves the quality of images and accuracy of the data obtained. Both left and right ventricular function can be assessed with this approach.
ii. The clinical context outlined is a classic description of (cardiac) syndrome X, i.e. anginal quality chest pain, a stress ECG showing ischaemic-like changes, and yet smooth normal arteries at angiography. In the absence of bundle branch block at rest or with exercise, it is most likely that the ventricular function will be normal (or super-normal) at rest and after pharmacological stress.

216 The question gives a typical case description of Takayasu's disease, a disorder characterised by an inflammatory process in the arterial wall, with degeneration and fibrosis of the media and adventitia. The patient is a young woman from the Orient. Initially, her illness was systemic and non-specific, with vague chest and abdominal discomfort and weight loss. Fever and arthralgia are also common at this stage, the inflammatory process itself contributing to the weight loss.

When she was examined, the physician thought she was shocked, but she was in fact 'pulseless'. The pronounced intimal proliferation characteristic of this disease had caused severe narrowing of the aortic arch branches, as well as of the lower aorta (i.e. Type 3 disease). Thus, her abdominal pain was actually due to mesenteric ischaemia. The day after admission, she had a cerebrovascular accident, due to involvement of the left common carotid artery, which proved fatal.

217 This patient has evidence of a muscular dystrophy and a cardiomyopathy. The death of her father at a very young age is a pointer that the condition is probably familial and that he died from a complication secondary to a cardiomyopathy. Familial dystrophies are often associated with dilated cardiomyopathy. There is considerable evidence of this in patients with Duchenne's and Becker's muscular dystrophies, which are X-linked, and in patients with Friedreich's ataxia, which is autosomal recessive. The latter can be associated with a hypertrophic cardiomyopathy. Female carriers of the X-linked muscular dystrophies and the infiltrative disorders may show evidence of cardiac abnormality, but it is less severe and at a later stage than in affected males.

Complications are those of all forms of dilated cardiomyopathy and include ventricular tachyarrythmias, systemic embolism and progressive cardiac failure. Treatment comprises conventional therapy for heart failure, anticoagulation to prevent emboli and amiodarone therapy to reduce the frequency of cardiac arrhythmias.

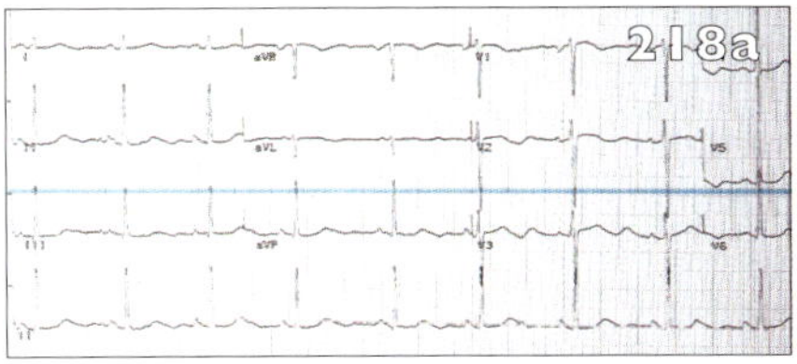

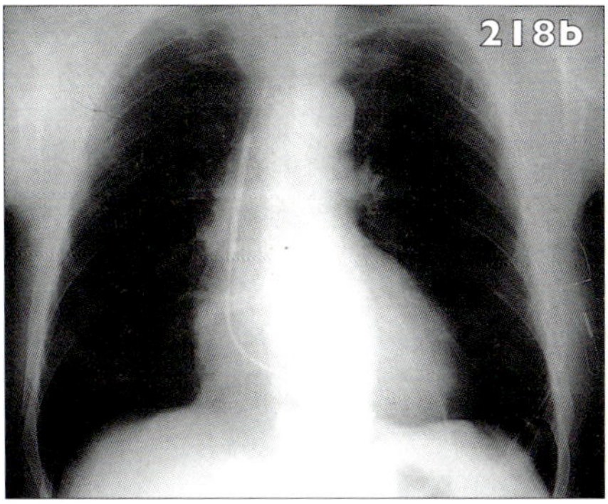

218 **i.** What is shown in **218a**?
ii. What is shown in **218b**?
iii. Briefly discuss the relationship between **218a** an **218b**.

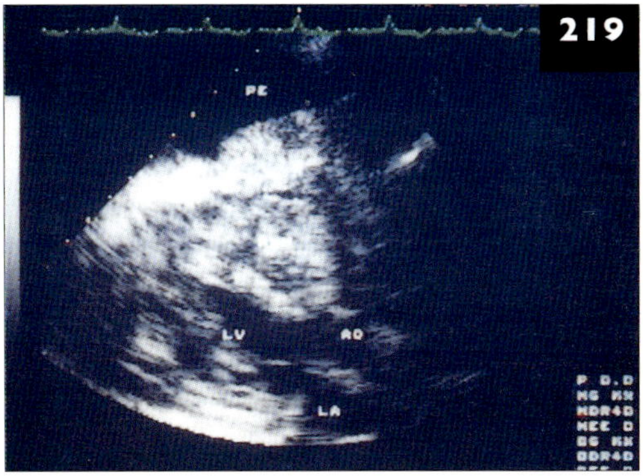

219 A 35-year-old male in-patient receiving chemotherapy for a non-Hodgkin's lymphoma underwent echocardiography for assessment of ventricular function prior to commencement of a more aggressive drug regimen. What incidental finding was made at echocardiography?

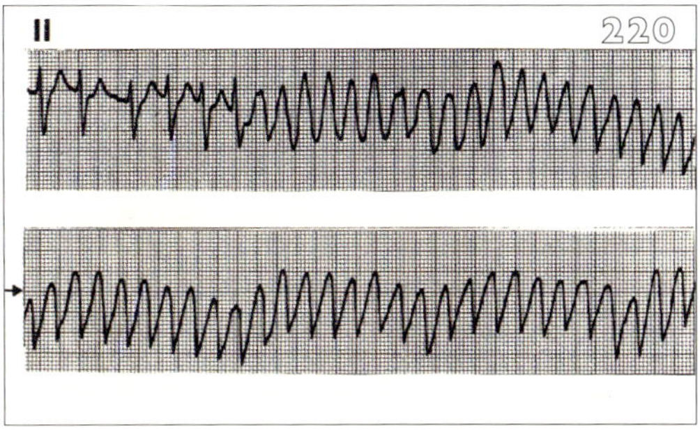

220 A 58-year-old man collapsed at the bus stop outside a hospital having visited a friend there. Two nurses were quickly on the scene, commenced cardiopulmonary resuscitation (CPR), and administered two 200 J DC shocks. The man was carried into the emergency department and the ECG trace obtained, as shown. What should be done next?

218 **i.** The ECG in slide **218a** shows prolongation of the QT interval.
ii. **218b** shows an automatic implantable cardioverter–defibrillator (AICD), located in the abdomen, with epicardial electrodes shown on the chest radiograph.
iii. The long QT shown in **218a** and the defibrillator implantation point to a diagnosis of long QT syndrome, a disorder probably due to abnormal functional efferent inputs to the heart, characterised by the development of lethal arrhythmias. The latter include torsades de pointes or polymorphic ventricular tachycardia which might degenerate into ventricular fibrillation. A family history of sudden cardiac death is common and two congenital forms are recognised. A long QT interval as well as congenital deafness characterise those with the Jervell and Lange-Nielsen syndromes (autosomal recessive), whereas deafness is not a feature of the Romano–Ward syndrome (autosomal dominant). Acquired prolongation of the QT interval is associated with drugs [especially class 1a, 1c, and class III anti-arrhythmics (mainly sotalol), lithium, and psychotropics], electrolyte disturbances (hypokalaemia, hypocalcaemia, and hypomagnesaemia), cardiac disorders (such as myocardial infarction and sick sinus syndrome), central nervous system injury (particularly in or around the right insula), toxins, and hypothermia. Beta-blockade appears to be protective and left cervical sympathectomy has been employed to a similar purpose. More recently, AICD has become established as an effective therapy.

219 The echocardiogram was obtained to measure left ventricular function before use of the cardiotoxic agent doxorubicin. However, during the echo, a mass was seen involving both the pericardium and left atrium. Neoplastic pericarditis is not rare, but is usually secondary to disseminated cancers of the lung, breast, or gastrointestinal tract. Lymphomas (Hodgkin's and non-Hodgkin's) account for about 15% of malignancies that metastasise to the heart. They occasionally present with pericardial effusion or even tamponade. However, a similar percentage of patients with lymphoma who eventually die and undergo post-mortem examination have evidence of cardiac metastatic disease. Thus, as here, involvement of the heart in metastatic disease may be silent; in contrast, pericardial involvement is likely to be manifest clinically.

220 The trace shows ventricular fibrillation. As early as feasible, a 200 J DC shock is given and repeated if successful defibrillation is not achieved; then a 360 J shock is tried. Competent cardiac massage (approximately 80 compressions/min) must be performed and ventilation commenced without delay (at five chest compressions to one breath). Ventilation can be mouth-to-mouth or mouth-to-nose initially, then Brooke airway or face mask/ambu-bag, but endotracheal intubation is used as soon as possible. Optimal venous access must be obtained – a central venous line ideally – to administer drugs. If the initial three shocks are unsuccessful, adrenaline 1 mg is given intravenously or, if venous access is not good, via the endotracheal tube at double the dose. Further 360 J shocks may be attempted at about every ten cycles of cardiopulmonary resuscitation and adrenaline administered with similar frequency. Anti-arrhythmics (initially lignocaine 100 mg followed, as necessary, by bretylium tosylate or amiodarone) are useful if the rhythm after defibrillation keeps reverting to ventricular tachycardia and/or ventricular fibrillation. The use of bicarbonate is now generally confined to circumstances of prolonged CPR (>15 minutes).

221 A 36-year-old man underwent surgery for the further management of his hypertension.
i. What was the underlying condition?
ii. How would you investigate this diagnostic possibility in a newly recognised hypertensive and what investigations are shown?
iii. Briefly describe how you would equip the anaesthetic trolley for this operation.

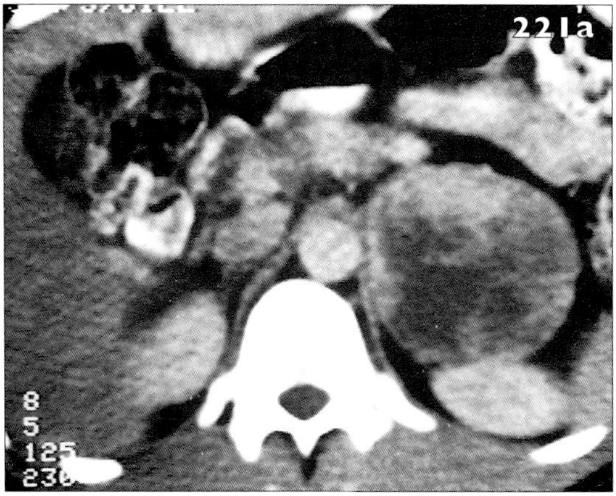

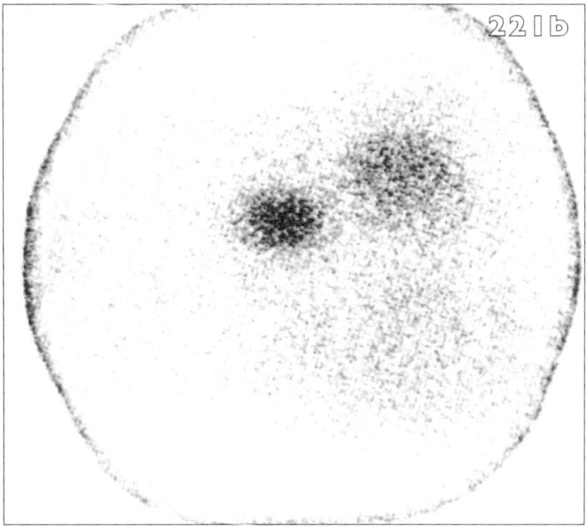

222 A 76-year-old woman who had been looked after by her family doctor for 'palpitations' and mild breathlessness for 3 years was admitted to the emergency department with a fractured radius. In view of her age and the possible need for general anaesthesia an ECG was performed and is illustrated above.
i. What is the most likely diagnosis?
ii. What further two test results would be helpful in confirming your view?

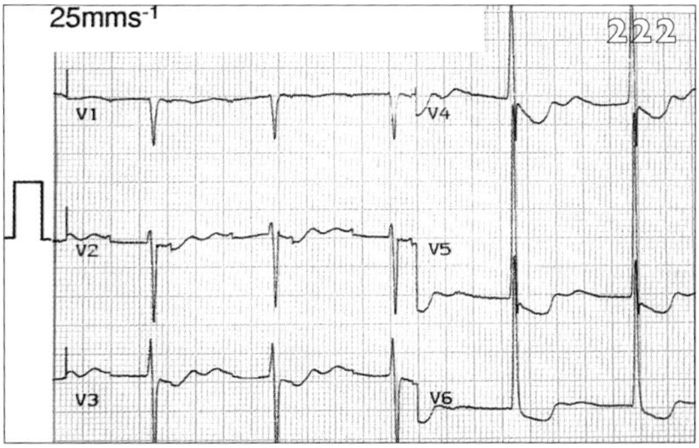

221 i. The patient had a phaeochromocytoma.
ii. Investigation of a patient who might have a phaeochromocytoma include measurement of urinary catecholamine metabolites [vanillylmandelic acid (VMA) and metanephrines] and (possibly) plasma catecholamines. **221a** is a tomogram of the abdomen, for anatomical localisation of the tumour, and **221b** is a scan using ^{131}I-metaiodobenzylguanidine (MIBG). The latter is useful for localisation of sites of active sympathetic tissue. CT and MR scans are the most valuable imaging techniques for the anatomical localisation of such tumours; regional venous sampling may also be needed for localisation of a small tumour outside the usual adrenal sites (paraganglionomas).
iii. The patient undergoing operative excision of a phaeochromocytoma must be well-prepared pre-operatively with separate alpha- (phenoxybenzamine or phentolamine) followed by beta-blocking agents (propranolol). During surgery, intra-arterial pressure monitoring is mandatory, to register rapidly the wide swings of blood pressure which can occur. The anaesthetic trolley should include intravenous labetolol, phentolamine, or nitroprusside (in case of marked hypertension), as well as fluids and noradrenaline in case of severe falls in blood pressure.

222 i. The ECG shows ST segment sag, with small T waves, but also prominent U waves; also, in the lateral chest leads, the ST segments have a 'reverse tick' morphology. The woman has hypokalaemia and possible digoxin excess. Originally, the family doctor had found her to have an irregularly irregular pulse, so diagnosed atrial fibrillation clinically and commenced therapy with digoxin without further investigation. The breathlessness had been assumed to be due to mild congestive cardiac failure and had responded well to a small regular dose of a loop diuretic. (On a background of digoxin toxicity, a range of arrhythmias may develop including ventricular bigeminy, salvoes of ventricular ectopics or ventricular tachycardia, junctional bradycardia, or second- or third-degree atrioventricular block.)
ii. Use of potassium-sparing diuretics in combination protects against digoxin toxicity and, indeed, reduces the myocardial digoxin concentration. Hypokalaemia is arrhythmogenic in its own right. The woman has been on diuretics for months, without a check on the electrolytes. Potassium levels must be checked. Digitalis levels do not need to be measured in patients with atrial fibrillation. Long-term diuretic usage can also deplete the body stores of magnesium (as can hypercalcaemia, hypoxia and hypothyroidism), which can predispose to digitalis toxicity. Serum magnesium levels are not especially helpful clinically, since most of the body's stocks are intracellular.

223 A 34-year-old West African woman presented with a 3 month history of increasing ankle oedema and abdominal distension. She had worked as a fish-farm administrator in Nigeria prior to moving to England 3 years previously. There was no history of cough, exertion dyspnoea, or orthopnoea. She was married with a 5-year-old daughter. She was a non-smoker and drank alcohol very occasionally.

Full blood count
Hb 12 g/dl
WCC 7 x 10^9/l (normal differential)
Platelets 300 x 10^9/l

Chest radiograph
Normal cardiac size and clear lung fields.

Urinalysis
Protein positive

ECG
Low QRS voltage and non-specific lateral T wave changes

On examination there was no evidence of pallor, jaundice, or lymphadenopathy. She had considerable pitting oedema of the legs, her heart rate was 100 irregularly irregular, blood pressure was 95/75 mmHg, JVP was elevated to the level of the ear lobes. On examination of the precordium the apex beat was not palpable. The heart sounds were soft, but there was an audible third heart sound. The chest was clear. Abdominal examination revealed hepatomegaly palpable 6 cm below the costal margin, as well as shifting dullness. The spleen was not palpable. Neurological examination and examination of the skin were normal. Investigations were as shown. What is the differential diagnosis and which test would you perform to differentiate between them?

224 This 45-year-old man was admitted to the coronary care unit complaining of chest pain at rest. What is the cause of his pain?

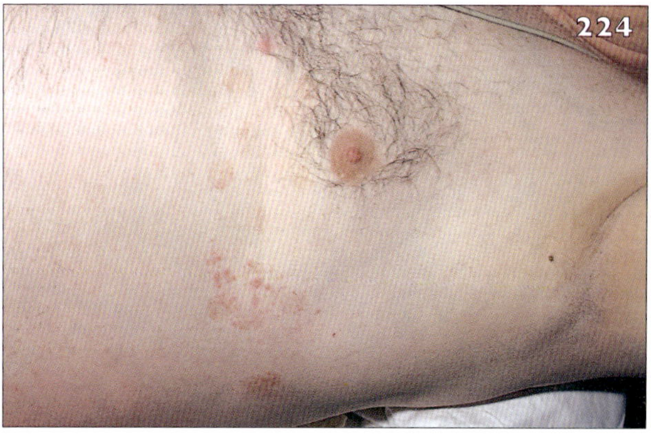

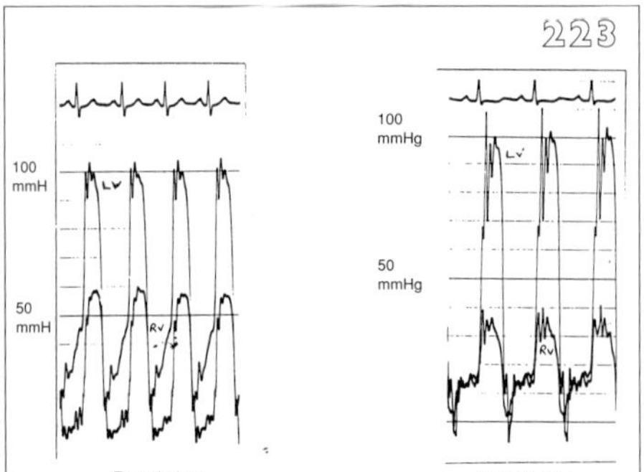

Restrictive pericarditis

Constrictive pericarditis

223 The differential diagnosis is between pericardial constriction and a restrictive cardiomyopathy. Both conditions present with predominantly right-sided cardiac failure and in both cases the heart size is often normal. Restrictive cardiomyopathy is common in West Africa and in this tropical variety eosinophilia may not be present, in contrast to the temperate variety where a marked eosinophilia is present (see **30**). Constrictive pericarditis in this case may be a sequel to previous tuberculous pericarditis (see **1**), but there is nothing in the history to suggest this. Some cases of constrictive pericarditis are idiopathic.

Echocardiography can occasionally differentiate between the two conditions. In constrictive pericarditis, the pericardium may be thickened. Cardiac catheterisation is often necessary before a definitive diagnosis can be made. The catheter traces of both restrictive cardiomyopathy and constrictive pericarditis are shown.

In constrictive pericarditis the disease affects the whole heart. The atrial pressures are high and equal with prominent x and y descents. The left ventricular end-diastolic pressure (LVEDP) is equal to the right ventricular end-diastolic pressure (RVEDP). The rapid filling in diastole produces a diastolic plateau wave form. In restrictive cardiomyopathy all of these changes apply with the main exception that the LVEDP and RVEDP vary widely. This is because the disease is patchy and often involves the right heart more than the left. The other main difference is that in constrictive pericarditis the early diastolic dip is below zero due to rapid filling, but in restrictive cardiomyopathy the early diastolic dip does not reach zero due to associated mitral and tricuspid regurgitation.

224 The man felt a severe continuous pain in his chest, although a more careful elicitation of the history would have revealed the burning character of the pain. The day following admission, the vesicles shown in the picture erupted. Their distribution in the left T4 dermatome enables a confident diagnosis of herpes zoster on clinical grounds alone, without the need for more detailed virological characterisation. In order to reduce the risk of post-herpetic neuralgia, treatment was commenced with oral acyclovir at a dose of 200 mg five times a day for a week and the situation resolved.

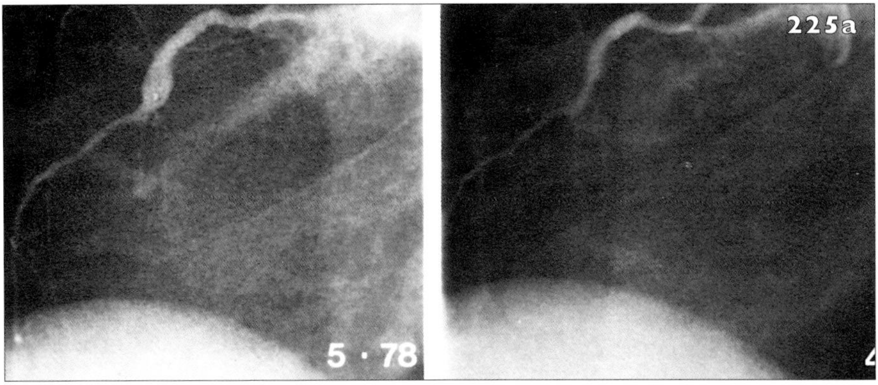

225a

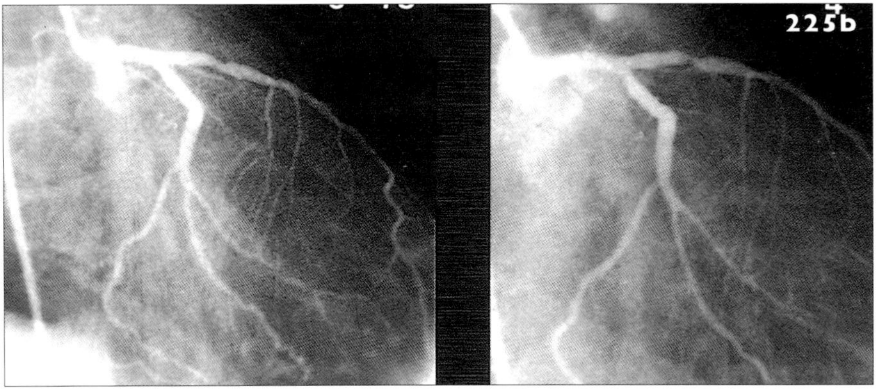
225b

225 This investigation was performed in a 40-year-old woman whose elder brother had died suddenly 5 years previously.

i. What does the picture show?

ii. Suggest the likely underlying diagnosis.

226 A 30-year-old woman who had an orthotopic cardiac transplant for dilated cardiomyopathy died 3 months later. 72 hours before her death she developed breathlessness and lethargy. List the two most likely causes of her death.

225 i. Angiography shows severe coronary atherosclerosis, including ostial stenosis. **ii.** Coronary disease of this severity in a young woman, with a family history of the premature and sudden death of a sibling, is suggestive of familial hypercholesterolaemia (FH). The woman had heterozygous FH and came to medical attention because of symptoms of angina pectoris. Studies of patients presenting with myocardial infarction show a ten-fold excess of FH patients. External signs of excessive cholesterol deposition, such as corneal arcus, xanthelasmata and tendon xanthomata are common. Coronary artery disease is characteristically severe and widespread, affecting the proximal as well as the distal coronary arteries. Usually all three epicardial vessels are affected and, in more than 30%, the left main stem is also significantly diseased.

226 The two most likely causes of death are either transplant rejection or infection due to immunosuppression. The most common causes of death following cardiac transplantation are rejection and infection. The third-commonest cause of mortality is coronary artery disease, which usually develops within 1 year of transplantation and is usually silent due to denervation of the transplanted heart. Rejection can present as fatigue, malaise, breathlessness, fever, depression, or personality change. The first episode of rejection usually occurs approximately 2 weeks after transplantation and over 80% of patients experience one or more episodes of rejection in the first year. The incidence of first episode rejection declines to a very low level (10/month/1000 patients) after 12 months. The exact reason for this is unclear but may be due to the development of immune tolerance. The diagnosis of rejection is made on endomyocardial biopsy which demonstrates infiltration of the myocardium with lymphocytes (see **141**). Treatment is with high-dose corticosteroids, usually intravenous methylprednisolone, in addition to cyclosporin and/or azathioprine, which the patient has usually commenced post-operatively. Antithymocyte globulin or OKT3, which is an antibody directed against CD3 lymphocytes, may be used for 5 or 10 days, respectively.

Opportunistic infection due to the immunosuppressive therapy used to prevent transplant rejection is the second most common cause of death in transplant patients. About 30% of patients experience an infectious episode within 3 months of transplantation and approximately 12% die. The organ involved most often is the lung and the most frequently implicated organism is cytomegalovirus. Overall, viruses cause 45% of infections, bacteria cause another 45% and fungi and protozoa account for the remainder. Mortality is highest with fungal infections.

Any transplant patient presenting with fever and breathlessness should have a full infection screen. Blood, urine and sputum are sent for viral, bacterial and fungal studies. In the absence of cardiac failure, breathlessness is most likely to be due to infection and is treated with anti-viral and broad spectrum antibiotics. Anti-fungal agents are commenced if the patient continues to deteriorate. In doubtful cases, cardiac biopsy is performed to resolve the differential diagnosis.

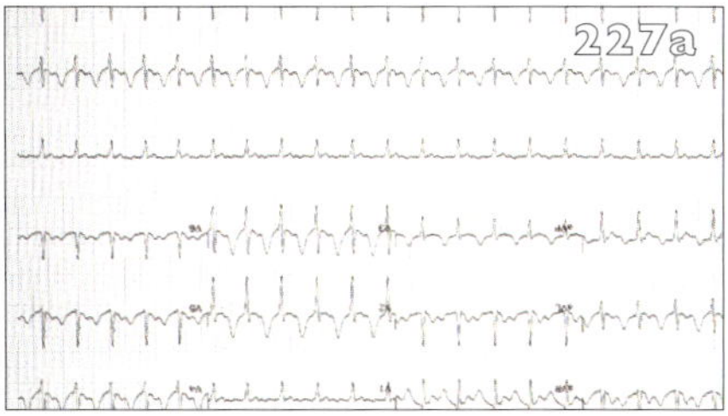

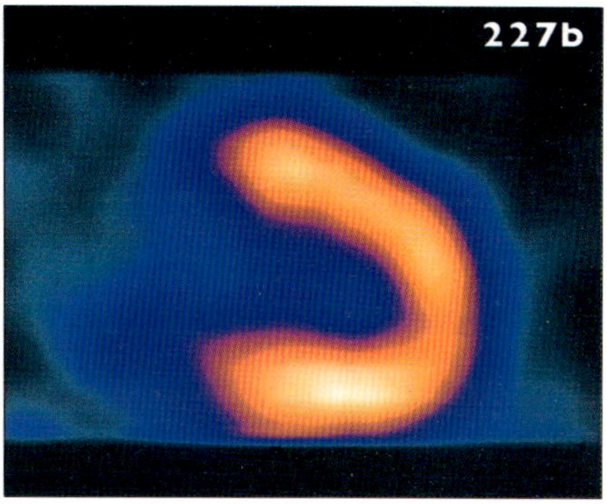

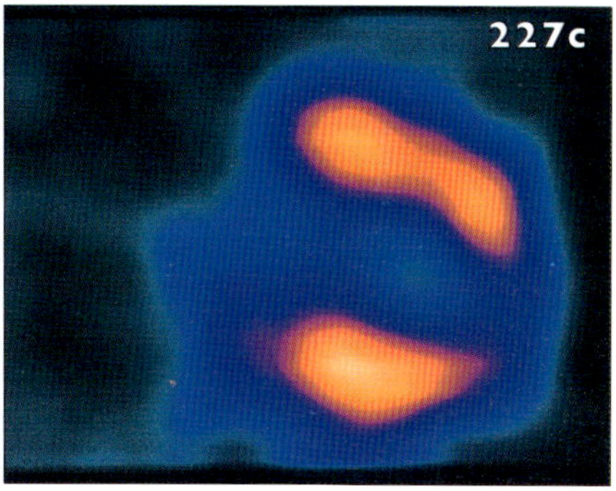

227 These results were obtained from a 55-year-old man with a 15-month history of effort-related breathlessness and chest tightness. He went on to have cardiac catheterisation and then a tight proximal stenosis of the diagonal branch of the left anterior descending coronary artery was discovered.

i. What can you determine from **227a**?

ii. What can you determine from **227b** and **227c** (obtained at rest and after pharmacological stress respectively)?

iii. Comment on the differences (if any) between your answers to **i** and **ii**.

228 A 69-year-old man who is 1.68 metres (5 feet 6 inches) tall and weighs 80 kg (195 pounds) is due to be discharged home one week after an uncomplicated inferior myocardial infarction. What advice are you going to give him? Thyroid function tests and blood glucose are normal.

227 i. 227a shows a normal electrocardiographic response to exercise with no diagnostic ST or T wave changes compatible with myocardial ischaemia.
ii. The thallium scans, **227b** and **227c**, show a reversible perfusion defect in the anteroapical region of the myocardium (i.e. the defect is absent at rest but demonstrable during pharmacological stress). The scan is consistent with reversible myocardial ischaemia.
iii. On the basis of the exercise ECG alone, Bayes' theorem would point to myocardial ischaemia being a likely cause of the breathlessness. However, the sensitivity of the exercise ECG is not greater than about 85% in the presence of coronary artery disease. The filling defect on the thallium scan would be consistent with a coronary artery lesion. Since the clinical picture is unclear, a stress echocardiogram may be of value in the non-invasive assessment of the motion of the anteroapical myocardium in real time at rest or during stress (exercise or pharmacological). In any case, coronary angiography was indicated because the patient came from a high-risk group (middle-aged male) and (most significantly) gave a typical history of angina.

228 Advice given to patients following myocardial infarction should be directed mainly towards reducing risk factors for coronary artery disease and allaying any anxieties which the patient may have. This man is clearly overweight and one of the main points to concentrate on would be dietary advice aimed at weight reduction and a low intake of saturated fats, bearing in mind the association between hypercholesterolaemia and coronary artery disease. He should be encouraged to exercise daily with a starting point of two short walks of approximately 15 minutes, increasing by 5 minutes weekly until he is walking between 2 and 4 miles daily. He should be advised regarding the use of GTN should he develop chest pain on exertion. Meta-analyses of the numerous trials performed on exercise following myocardial infarction suggest some benefit with a reduction of up to 25% in post-myocardial infarction mortality. Exercise following myocardial infarction increases the ischaemic threshold as well as serum HDL cholesterol levels and aids weight reduction. Although mild-to-moderate exercise is beneficial, vigorous sport may be contra-indicated.

He should stop smoking if this is applicable. Similarly, co-existing diabetes mellitus and hypertension should be checked regularly and controlled. Alcohol in moderation, i.e. two units daily, is perfectly satisfactory, but higher quantities, particularly of beer (which is high in calories), should be discouraged.

If he holds a licence for passenger-carrying vehicles, he should refrain from driving for 1 month. To re-apply for a licence to drive heavy vehicles, he must demonstrate an ability to exercise for 9 minutes according to the Bruce protocol or equivalent without any inducible myocardial ischaemia.

Aeroplane travel is not advisable for the first month. Sexual intercourse is best avoided for 6 weeks and a passive role should initially be encouraged on resuming his sex life.

Finally, the patient should be made aware of symptoms which may be attributable to cardiovascular disease, in order to maximise the patient's autonomy.

Appendix

	Adult
Venae cavae	
Mean	2–8
Right atrium	
a wave	3–6
v wave	1–4
Mean	1–5
Right ventricle	
Systolic	20–30
End diastolic	2–7
Pulmonary artery	
Systolic	16–30
Diastolic	4–13
Mean	9–18
Pulmonary capillary wedge position	4.5–12
Left atrium	
a wave	4–14
v wave	6–16
Mean	6–11
Left ventricle	
Systolic	90–140
End diastolic	6–12
Aorta	
Systolic	90–140
Diastolic	70–90
Mean	70–110

Table 1. Range of normal intracardiac and intravascular pressures (mHg) in adults at rest in the supine position. (Adapted from Geigy Scientific Tables, CIBA-GEIGY, 1990.)

	Number	*Mean*	*Range*
Right atrium			
Mean	44	1	–2–6
Right ventricle			
Systolic	44	24	15–37
End diastolic	44	3	0–8
Pulmonary artery			
Systolic	44	20	12–35
Diastolic	44	7	3–12
Mean	44	11	7–18
Left atrium			
Mean	9	6	2–14
Left ventricle			
Systolic	21	100	72–103
End diastolic	21	7	3–14
Peripheral artery			
Systolic	37	108	84–150
Diastolic	37	64	50–83
Mean	37	81	67–105

Table 2. Intracardiac and intravascular pressures (mmHg)in children (aged 1 week to 16 years) at rest in the supine position. (Adapted from Geigy Scientific Tables, CIBA-GEIGY, 1990.)

Index

Numbers refer to question and answer numbers

Abscess, 49, 182
Acromegaly, 2
Adenosine, 62, 123
Adrenal adenoma, 47, 178
Adrenalitis, tuberculous, 173
Alcoholic cardiomyopathy, 61
Amiodarone, 109, 148, 208
Amyloidosis (AL), 74
Anaemia, haemolytic, 86
Aneurysm
- aortic, *see* Aortic aneurysm
- left ventricular, 94
- mycotic, 183
Angina, variant (Prinzmetal's), 196
Angiography, 28, 45, 122, 150
Angiotensin-converting enzyme (ACE) inhibitor, 137, 168, 195
Ankylosing spondylitis, 57
Aorta
- coarctation, 25, 46, 91, 99, 150
- descending, stenosis, 150
- ulcerated plaques, 202
Aortic aneurysm
- ascending aorta, 37, 108
- Dacron patch site, 25
- syphilitic, 108
- thoracic, 27, 72
Aortic arch, narrowing, 216
Aortic dissection, 42, 143, 210
Aortic knuckle, 91, 99, 142
Aortic regurgitation, 6, 57, 88, 92, 101, 200
Aortic root dissection, 42
Aortic stenosis, 34, 39, 72, 102, 116, 161, 170, 179
Aortic valve
- abscess, 182
- bicuspid, 39, 180
- calcification, 39, 170
- congenital abnormality, 39
- incompetence, 88
- prosthesis/replacement, 86, 104, 170
Aortitis, 108
Aortography, 57, 150
Apexcardiogram (ADC), 207
Arteriography, 66, 70, 137, 172
Ascites, 5
Atherectomy catheter, 105
Atrial arrhythmia, re-entrant, 35
Atrial fibrillation (AF), 50, 55, 77, 109, 168, 186
- chronic, digoxin in, 81
- 'lone', 77
- paroxysmal, 147
Atrial flutter, 35, 211
Atrial myxoma, 78, 83
Atrial premature beats (APBs), 166
Atrial septal defect (ASD), 45, 95, 103, 128
- ostium primum, 65, 95, 154, 203
- ostium secundum, 23, 64, 203
Atrial tachyarrhythmia, 35, 84
Atrioventricular block, 96, 167
- first-degree, 90, 135
- second-degree (Mobitz Types I/II), 44, 93, 185, 204
- third-degree, 139, 195
Atrioventricular canal, partial, 65, 95, 154, 203
Atrioventricular dissociation, 56
Atrioventricular nodal re-entrant tachycardia (AVNRT), 59, 62
Atrioventricular node, conduction pathways, 60
Atrioventricular tachycardia, 59, 211
Atrium, single, 119
Austin Flint murmur, 88, 92, 101
Automatic implantable cardioverter–defibrillator (AICD), 29, 218

Back pain, 57, 108
Balloon septostomy, 45
Bernoulli equation, 102
Biventricular failure, 5, 190
Bjork–Shiley mechanical valve, 104
Bradycardia, 84, 160, 175, 206
Brockenbrough phenomenon, 68
Bruce protocol exercise test, 186
Buerger's test, 191
Bundle branch block
- left (LBBB), 10, 93, 155, 161, 167
- right (RBBB), 64, 65, 133, 154, 197
Bundle of Kent, 60

Calcium antagonists, 85
Cannon waves, 163
Carcinoid syndrome, 171
Cardiac catheterisation, 20, 65, 68, 71, 75, 116, 162, 200
Cardiac failure, 1, 5, 80, 190, 192
- congestive, 5, 81, 163
Cardiac injury, 134
Cardiac tamponade, 36, 163
Cardiac transplantation, 80, 141, 226
Cardiomegaly, 64, 206
Cardiomyopathy, 9
- alcoholic, 61
- dilated, 217
- HIV, 144
- hypertrophic, 3, 68, 181, 212
- peripartum, 19
- restrictive, 30, 223
Cardiopulmonary bypass, 41
Cardiopulmonary resuscitation (CPR), 220
Cardioversion, 109
Cardioverter defibrillators, automatic implantable, 29, 218
Carotid artery, left common, stenosis, 76
Chagas' disease, 167
Cholesterol embolus, retinal, 41
Chondroectodermal dysplasia, 119
Chronic obstructive airways disease, 32, 149, 199
Circumflex artery, 172
Claudication, intermittent, 137
Clubbing, fingers/toes, 11, 152

Coal worker's pneumoconiosis, 199
Coarctation of aorta, 25, 46, 91, 99, 150
Cocaine, 122
Computed tomography (CT) scans, 1, 183, 210
Congenital heart disease, 11, 28, 128
Congestive cardiac failure, 5, 81, 163
Conn's syndrome, 178
Coronary arteriography/angiography, 66, 172, 201
Coronary artery
- atherectomy, 105
- congenital abnormalities, 38
- dissection, 162
- ectasia, 159
- restenosis, 66, 105, 213
- spasm, 122, 196
- stenosis, 24, 122, 176
- subacute occlusion, 184
- tortuous/dilated, 72
- ulcerated plaques, 202
Coronary artery bypass grafting (CABG), 24, 33, 41, 121, 132, 193
Coronary artery disease (CAD), 123, 136, 148, 155, 156, 187, 225
Coronary stents, 66
Cor pulmonale, 32, 149
Cortisol, elevated, 47
Creatine kinase (CK), 48
Cyanosis, 11, 45, 90, 128, 142

Dacron patch grafting, 25
Deep vein thrombosis, 193
Dextrocardia, 153
Diabetes insipidus, 47
Diabetes mellitus, 120, 131, 191
Digitalis, 81
Digital subtraction angiography, 76
Digoxin, 81, 222
Digoxin toxicity, 59, 222
Disseminated intravascular coagulation (DIC), 67
Diuretics, 146, 214, 222
Doppler echocardiography, 21, 65, 130
- continuous-wave, 6, 21, 55, 102, 203
- pulsed-wave, 55, 102
Doppler study, colour-flow, 130, 203
Down syndrome, 157
Doxorubicin, cardiotoxicity, 190, 219
Drug abusers, 8, 183
Duckett–Jones diagnostic criteria, 13, 82
Ductus arteriosus, patent, 11, 28
Dystrophia myotonica, 17

Ebstein's anomaly, 211
Echocardiography, 34, 106
- 2D, 9, 54, 97, 168, 169, 180
- M mode, 7, 12, 83, 101, 107, 143, 144
- stress, 123, 227
- transoesophageal, 42, 182, 210
- transthoracic, 63, 210
- *see also* Doppler echocardiography
Ectopic beats, 166, 198
Eisenmenger's syndrome, 90
Electrocardiogram (ECG)
- ambulatory, 84, 205
- d-wave, 109
- J waves, 69
- PR interval prolonged, 135
- QRS complex changes, 10, 44, 56, 62, 133, 208
- QT interval prolongation, 146, 214, 218
- ST segment depression, 179, 184, 187, 205
- ST segment elevation, 4, 120, 195, 196
'Electromechanical dissociation', 124
Ellis–van Creveld syndrome, 119
Embolectomy, 31, 63
Endocarditis
- infective, *see* Infective endocarditis
- Libman–Sacks, 145
Endocardium, ulceration, 49
Endomyocardial biopsy, 141
Endomyocardial fibrosis (EMF), tropical, 30
Eosinophilia, 223
Erythema chronicum migrans, 96
Erythema marginatum, 13
Erythema nodosum, 18
Exercise testing, 79, 186, 212, 227
- contraindications, 34, 187

Fallot's tetralogy, 71
Familial hypercholesterolaemia (FH), 156, 202, 225
Flushing, 171

Grave's disease, 50
Gum hypertrophy, 85

Haemochromatosis, 165
Haemolytic anaemia, microangiopathic, 86
Haemosiderin, 129
Heart, right-to-left shunt, 71
Heart block
- complete, 44, 59, 96, 111, 115
- *see also* Atrioventricular block; Bundle branch block
Heart murmurs, 142
- Austin Flint, 88, 92, 101
- diastolic, 83, 92, 186
- late systolic, 50, 68, 87, 212
- 'machinery', 28
- pan-systolic, 53, 130, 168
- systolic, 23, 46, 90, 112, 161, 169, 186
Heart sounds, second, splitting, 161, 170, 203
Heparin, 193
Herpes zoster, 224
Hilar lymphadenopathy, 18
His–Purkinje disease, 17
HIV infection, 144
Holter electrocardiography, 84, 205
5-Hydroxytryptamine, 171
Hyperaldosteronism, 47
Hypercholesterolaemia, 52, 127
- familial, 156, 202, 225
Hypertension, 2, 43, 89, 174, 178, 221
- pulmonary, *see* Pulmonary hypertension
Hypertensive encephalopathy, 89
Hyperthyroidism, 50
Hypertrophic cardiomyopathy (HCM), 3, 68, 181, 212
Hypoadrenalism, 173
Hypokalaemia, 47, 146, 214, 222
Hypotension, 4, 160, 169, 173
Hypothermia, 69
Hypothyroidism, 189, 206

Idiopathic hypertrophic subaortic stenosis (IHSS), *see* Hypertrophic cardiomyopathy
Iliofemoral embolism, 63
Immunosuppression, 226
Infections, opportunistic, 226
Infective endocarditis, 8, 63, 78, 125, 182, 183, 194, 209
- acute pyogenic, 49
- surgery indications, 114
Intra-aortic balloon counterpulsation, 117
Iron oxide, inhalation, 126

James fibres, 60
Janeway lesions, 194
Jervell syndrome, 214, 218
Jugular venous pressure (JVP), 130, 163

Kartagener's syndrome, 153
Kerley B lines, 15
Kussmaul's sign, 163

Lange–Nielsen syndrome, 214, 218
Left anterior descending (LAD) coronary artery, 155, 172
- grafting, 121
- stenosis, 24, 122
Left anterior hemiblock, 133
Left atrial enlargement, 9, 15, 31, 107, 110, 129
Left atrial myxoma, 78, 83
Left atrial pressure, 103
Left coronary artery, 38, 172
- main, stenosis, 136
Left internal mammary artery (LIMA) graft, 121
Left ventricular aneurysm, 94
Left ventricular dilatation, 9, 15, 61, 94, 101, 168
Left ventricular end-diastolic pressure (LVEDP), 75, 116, 223
Left ventricular end-diastolic/systolic dimensions, 144, 168
Left ventricular hypertrophy, 30, 34, 88, 174
Left ventricular infarction, 36
Left ventricular premature beat, 140
Left ventricular pressure, 39
Left ventricular rupture, 36
Left ventricular thrombosis, 30, 97
Lenègre's disease, 111
Leukaemia, acute, 190
Libman–Sacks endocarditis, 145
Long QT syndrome, 218
Low density lipoprotein (LDL), excess, 156
Lown–Ganong–Levine syndrome, 60
Lung, hyperinflation, 32
Lutembacher's syndrome, 103
Lyme disease, 96
Lymphoma, metastases in heart, 219

Magnesium, 146, 222
Magnetic resonance imaging (MRI), 25, 95
Mahaim fibres, 60
Marfan's syndrome, 143
Mitral paravalvar abscess, 182
Mitral regurgitation, 65, 75, 114, 116, 130, 145, 154, 168
Mitral stenosis, 20, 55, 103, 129, 138, 186, 188, 200
- atrial myxoma *vs*, 78, 83
Mitral valve
- abnormal motion of leaflets, 68
- calcification, 15
- floppy, 87
- fluttering, 101
- prolapse, 50, 73, 87, 116
- prosthesis/replacement, 51, 114, 188
- rheumatic disease, 12, 15, 110, 168, 188
- St Jude prosthesis, stenosis, 188
- thickening of leaflets, 12
- vegetation, 63
Mixed mitral valve disease, 31
Muscular dystrophy, 217
Mycotic aneurysm, 183
Myocardial dystrophy, 17
Myocardial fibrosis, 18
Myocardial hypertrophy, 181, 200
Myocardial infarction
- advice after, 228
- anterior, 16, 48, 67, 93, 97, 120, 131, 207
- anteroapical, 26
- complications, 36, 130, 140
- inferior, 21, 125, 176, 195, 200
- inferolateral, 4
- painless ('silent'), 120, 131, 205
- posterior, 176
- subendocardial anterolateral, 184
Myocardial ischaemia, 120, 135, 179, 205, 208, 227
Myocardial necrosis, 48, 141
Myocarditis, 9, 19, 40
Myocardium, inflammatory infiltrate, 19, 40, 141
Myxoedema, 189
Myxoma, atrial, 78, 83

Ostium primum atrial septal defect, 65, 95, 154, 203
Ostium secundum atrial septal defect, 23, 64, 203

Pacemakers/pacing, 56, 58, 139, 175
- dual chamber, 139, 158, 160
- single chamber, 118, 139
Pacemaker syndrome, 58
Paget's disease of bone, 192
Palpitations, 54, 59, 166
Parkinsonian tremor, 115
Patent ductus arteriosus, 11, 28
Pectus excavatum, 100
Percutaneous transluminal coronary angioplasty (PTCA), 66, 213
Pericardial effusion, 7, 30, 106, 151
'Pericardial knock', 113
Pericardial tamponade, 7
Pericarditis, 106
- constrictive, 1, 113, 163, 223
- tuberculous, 151
Pericardium, calcification, 1
Peripartum cardiomyopathy, 19
Peripheral vascular disease, 191
Phaeochromocytoma, 174, 221
Polyarteritis nodosa, 125
Polyuria, 47
Postural hypotension, 173
Potassium ferricyanide stains, 165
Pregnancy, 19, 128, 169

Prinzmetal's angina, 196
Pseudoxanthoma elasticum, 73
Pulmonary artery, post-stenotic dilatation, 177
Pulmonary artery occlusion, 14
Pulmonary artery pressure, raised, 20, 75, 200
Pulmonary balloon valvoplasty, percutaneous, 112
Pulmonary capillary wedge pressure, raised, 20, 75, 116, 200
Pulmonary embolism, acute, 14, 193
Pulmonary hypertension, 32, 85, 110, 128, 142, 149, 199
– secondary, 20, 64
Pulmonary oedema, non-cardiogenic, 126
Pulmonary plethora, 64
Pulmonary valve stenosis, 71, 112, 177
'Pulseless' disease (Takayasu's), 216

Radial–femoral arterial pulse delay, 91, 150
Rectal temperature, 69
Renal artery stenosis, 137
Respiratory failure, type II, 149
Restenosis, coronary arteries, 66, 105, 213
Retina, cholesterol embolus, 41
Retinal haemorrhage, 131
Retinopathy, 89, 131
Rhabdomyolysis, 52
Rheumatic fever, 13, 82, 107, 188
– mitral valve disease, 12, 15, 110, 168, 188
Rib notching, 91, 99
Right atrial dilatation, 32, 95
Right atrial pressure, increased, 20, 211
Right coronary artery, 24, 70, 176, 213
Right ventricular dilatation, 15, 32, 95
Right ventricular end-diastolic pressure (RVEDP), 223
Right ventricular failure, 1,.5
Right ventricular hypertrophy, 64, 90, 110, 142, 149, 177, 199
Right ventricular infarction, 4, 21
Right ventricular pressure, raised, 20, 71, 75, 200
Romano–Ward syndrome, 214, 218
Rotablator, 105
Roth spots, 125, 194

St Jude mechanical valve prosthesis, 188
Saphenous vein bypass graft, 33
Sarcoidosis, 18
Scleroderma, 43
Sick sinus syndrome, 84, 139
Single photon emission computed tomography (SPECT), 155, 215
Sinoatrial disease, 175
Sinus bradycardia, 69
Sinus tachycardia, 50
Sinus of Valsalva, 38, 143
Situs inversus, 153
Staphylococcus aureus, 8, 49
Starr–Edwards prosthesis, 51, 86, 104
Statin drugs, 52, 127
Stokes–Adams attacks, 17, 58, 111
Streptococcal infections, 13, 82
Stroke, 77, 147, 216
Stroke volume, increased, 169
Sudden cardiac death, 38, 205, 218
Superior vena cava obstruction, 37
Supraventricular tachycardia, 62
Swan-Ganz catheterisation, 130
Syndrome X, 215
Syphilitic aortitis, 108
Systemic lupus erythematosus (SLE), 145
Systemic sclerosis, 43

Tabes dorsalis, 108
Tachycardia, *see specific types of tachycardia*
'Tachy–Brady' syndrome, 84
Takayasu's disease, 216
Thallium scans, 155, 227
Thiazide diuretics, 146
Thrombolytic therapy, 14, 195
Tilt-table testing, 160
Toe infarction, 31
Toes, clubbing, 11
Torsades de pointes, 214
Transposition of great vessels, 45
Tricuspid regurgitation, 21, 65, 75, 211
Tricuspid valve displacement, 211
Trypanosomiasis, American (Chagas' disease), 167
Tuberculosis, 151, 173
'Tumour plop', 83
Turner's syndrome, 46

Valsalva manoeuvre, 32, 164
Vasculitis, 125
Vasovagal syndrome, 'malignant', 160
Ventricular bigemini, 59
Ventricular extrasystole, 198
Ventricular fibrillation, 220
Ventricular pacing/pacemakers, 56, 58, 118, 139, 175
Ventricular septal defect (VSD), 4, 16, 22, 71, 90, 130, 142
– restrictive, 53
– traumatic, 134
Ventricular septal hypertrophy, 3
Ventricular tachycardia, 29, 98, 146, 179, 198, 208, 212
– polymorphic, 214
Ventricular thrombosis, 30, 97
Ventriculo-arterial discordance, 45
Ventriculogram, radionuclide multi-gated (MUGA), 215
Viral myocarditis, 9, 40

Wenckebach AV block, 204
Williams' syndrome, 72
Wolff–Parkinson–White syndrome, 60, 62, 109